Resistance Training Instruction

SECOND EDITION

Everett Aaberg

Director of Fitness Services and Co-Owner
TELOS Fitness Center
Dallas, Texas

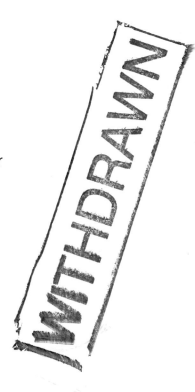

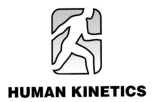

HUMAN KINETICS

Library of Congress Cataloging-in-Publication Data

Aaberg, Everett, 1963-
  Resistance training instruction / Everett Aaberg. -- 2nd ed.
    p. cm.
  Includes bibliographical references and index.
  ISBN-13: 978-0-7360-6403-3 (soft cover)
  ISBN-10: 0-7360-6403-6 (soft cover)
  1. Weight training. 2. Exercise. 3. Personal trainers. I. Title.
  GV546.A237 2007
  613.7'1--dc22

                    2006027900

ISBN-10: 0-7360-6403-6
ISBN-13: 978-0-7360-6403-3

Acquisitions Editor: Martin Barnard
Developmental Editor: Kevin Matz
Assistant Editor: Laura Koritz
Copyeditor: Jan Feeney
Proofreader: Pam Johnson
Indexer: Susan Hernandez
Graphic Designers: Bob Reuther and Nancy Rasmus
Graphic Artist: Tara Welsch
Photo Manager: Laura Fitch
Cover Designer: Keith Blomberg
Photographer (cover and interior): Sarah Ritz
Art Manager: Kelly Hendren
Illustrators: Figure 6.1 by Kareema McLendon-Foster; muscle drawings on pages 108-245 by Hoc K. Kho, Brian F. Wilson, Shannon Bean, and Merideth A. Philips/Nucleus Medical Art, Inc.; all other illustrations by Scott Beckley
Printer: Custom Color Graphics

Human Kinetics books are available at special discounts for bulk purchase. Special editions or book excerpts can also be created to specification. For details, contact the Special Sales Manager at Human Kinetics.

Printed in the United States of America   10 9 8 7 6 5 4 3 2 1

Human Kinetics
Web site: www.HumanKinetics.com

United States: Human Kinetics
P.O. Box 5076
Champaign, IL 61825-5076
800-747-4457
e-mail: humank@hkusa.com

Canada: Human Kinetics
475 Devonshire Road Unit 100
Windsor, ON N8Y 2L5
800-465-7301 (in Canada only)
e-mail: orders@hkcanada.com

Europe: Human Kinetics
107 Bradford Road
Stanningley
Leeds LS28 6AT, United Kingdom
+44 (0) 113 255 5665
e-mail: hk@hkeurope.com

Australia: Human Kinetics
57A Price Avenue
Lower Mitcham, South Australia 5062
08 8372 0999
e-mail: liaw@hkaustralia.com

New Zealand: Human Kinetics
Division of Sports Distributors NZ Ltd.
P.O. Box 300 226 Albany
North Shore City
Auckland
0064 9 448 1207
e-mail: info@humankinetics.co.nz

Resistance Training Instruction

SECOND EDITION

Contents

Preface **vi**

Part I   Human Movement and Adaptation

1

Anatomical Design and Function 3

Discusses the control system, the active system, and the passive system.

2

Joint Mechanics 19

Details the joint movements and muscle mechanics for each of the three planes of motion.

3

Resistance Training Adaptations 29

Presents resistance exercise adaptations that are related to improving the performance of the body and the enhancement of biomotor abilities.

Part II   Technique and Programming

4

Resistance Training Technique 53

Clarifies specific points of proper exercise technique, including exercise motion, alignment, positioning, stabilization, tempo, and breathing.

5

Resistance Exercise Selection. 67

Shows how different factors affect the selection of exercises: determining goals, targeting desired movements and muscle groups, and comparing the risk versus benefit of an exercise.

6 Resistance Exercise Program Design .. 81

Shows how to use the principles of exercise selection to create a comprehensive and effective program.

Part III Exercises

7 Core and Trunk Exercises. 107

Exercises for the core and trunk muscles.

8 Compound Lower-Body Exercises 139

Compound exercises for the pelvic, hip, and leg muscles.

9 Isolated Lower-Body Exercises 165

Isolated exercises for the pelvic, hip, and leg muscles.

10 Upper-Body Pushing Exercises. 197

Exercises for the scapular, shoulder, elbow, and wrist muscles responsible for pushing actions.

11 Upper-Body Pulling Exercises. 219

Exercises for the scapular, shoulder, elbow, and wrist muscles responsible for pulling actions.

Bibliography **246** I Index **247** I About the Author **250**

Preface

The mission of *Resistance Training Instruction, Second Edition,* is to provide fitness professionals and strength coaches with the most critical information they will need in order to understand and teach others how to select, modify, and perform resistance training exercises based on the structure and true function of the human body. This text also presents principles of biomechanics and realistic methods of organizing resistance training exercises into actual periodized training routines and programs that will help to improve the performance, conditioning, aesthetics, and overall health of the athletes and clients they train.

The human body is extremely complex in its design and even more so in its integrated function of the various systems. Research is confirming how all systems, including digestive, endocrine, lymphatic, and cardiorespiratory systems, are linked to and affected by the health and function of the skeletal, muscular, and neurological systems responsible for production and control of all movement. Therefore, despite all that we already know about the benefits of physical fitness, I believe we are only beginning to scratch the surface of how important regular exercise is to maintaining overall health and well-being.

However, it is not within the scope of this book to present such complex information but rather to maintain the focus on presenting training methods and techniques that will enhance the conditioning and biomotor abilities of the human body. It is also the aim of this text to condense and simplify the vast amounts of information that encompass the in-depth studies of anatomy, kinesiology, physiology, neurology, motor development, physics, and biomechanics.

Fortunately, as complex as the human body is internally, it was also designed to perform fairly simple general movement patterns in order to interact within the earth's environment and function with gravity. Given these facts, it is possible to present specific movement strategies and techniques that are safe and effective for improving human performance in a simplified and concise manner.

By design, only a carefully selected sampling of some of the most effective exercises for training the major muscles and muscular subsystems of the body are presented in this book. However, by first understanding the principles also presented, a proficient trainer should be able to modify and create countless exercise variations and organize them into effective training programs to meet any client's or athlete's specific training needs and goals. Many of these training principles, exercises, and techniques are time proven and have been used by numerous top trainers and strength coaches around the globe. My own staff of trainers and therapists at the TELOS Fitness Center also incorporate them on a daily basis in order to improve the strength, endurance, mobility, stability, speed, power, agility, and aesthetics of our clients and athletes. This book also serves as an instructional text for several fitness education organizations as well as numerous colleges and universities. I hope you will find the information and tools provided in this book valuable and learn to apply them with confidence and passion to help you and your clients reach your goals and theirs.

Human Movement and Adaptation

This book is directed toward providing you—as a fitness professional, personal trainer, or strength coach—with valuable information that will help you improve your clients' and athletes' performance, appearance, and overall health through the use of resistance training exercise. Part I provides the most pertinent information about how the human body is designed to move and about the beneficial adaptations that will result in response to resistance training.

This part first presents the essentials of the structure and true function of the human movement systems. It will help you understand how the body is designed to move as a linked kinetic chain through the integrated work of the skeletal, muscular, and neural systems as opposed to simply seeing movement as a collection of isolated joint and muscle actions. You will learn how to select exercise movements and use specific techniques to improve your clients' movement performance as safely as possible, which is a topic presented in part II of this book.

Part I provides critical information related to the adaptations that your clients can achieve through the use of resistance training. The focus is directed toward the potential outcomes versus the actual physiological processes of adaptation. This means that the emphasis is on biomotor development such as what is required for enhancing strength, endurance, stability, mobility, speed, power, and agility. Other often-desired adaptations relating to aesthetics, such as increased muscle size and decreased body fat, are also covered here to give you direction in helping clients and athletes look better as well as perform better.

Anatomical Design and Function

It is logical to assume that any resistance training exercise or technique should be based on the actual structure and true function of the human body. Therefore it would be wise to first understand how the body is constructed before beginning resistance training or prescribing exercises or techniques to others. The human body is a sophisticated machine with a large number of components that combine to produce an infinite variety of postures and movements. These components function together as interdependent systems and subsystems.

A contemporary view of functional anatomy presents the body as composed of three general interdependent systems: the passive system, the active system, and the control system. All three must work together synergistically to produce motion or to provide stability at every joint of the body. Therefore, since any exercise requires a certain combination of both movement and stability, each will impress a unique training effect on all three major systems, not just the targeted muscle. Furthermore, efficient exercise selection and technique are critical for achieving any desired effect, because every exercise performed not only will affect the body's "hardware," such as the joints and muscles, but also leave an imprint on the "software," or neural systems. The resistance training exercises and techniques selected and performed will literally program the body for success or for failure in reaching its potential.

The basic integrated relationships of the three major systems are depicted in figure 1.1. As the body begins to perform any movement, whether voluntarily or through reflex actions, the control (or sensorimotor) system issues commands to the active (or muscular) system to initiate a concert of muscular actions complete with the recommended force outputs necessary for stabilizing and moving the passive (or skeletal) system in order to produce the desired movement. Even automated actions of the body, such as breathing, coughing, sneezing, or flinching, require specific integrated actions of all three systems. We present the components and the movement-related responsibilities of each system, beginning with the passive (skeletal) system, followed by the active (muscular) system, and then tie those together with the control (sensorimotor) system.

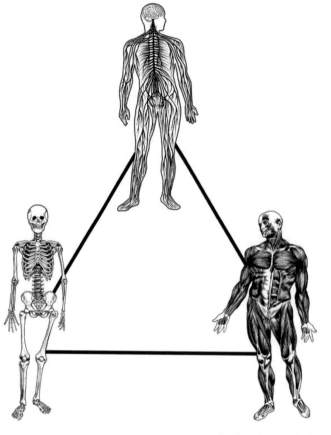

Control (sensorimotor) system

Passive (skeletal) system

Active (muscular) system

Figure 1.1 The three systems of human movement.

Passive System

The passive system is composed of the skeleton, joints, and associated connective tissues. It is termed *passive* because no independent action associated with movement can be accomplished by this system. It is a reactive system that totally relies on either internal forces produced by the neuromuscular system to provide for active movement or external forces such as gravity that can produce passive movement if not resisted.

Skeleton

At birth the human body has approximately 270 bones, some of which are designed to fuse during growth. By the time humans reach full growth, the skeleton normally consists of only 206 bones that are connected in such a way as to enable the body to best function and interact with its environment. The skeleton performs three main mechanical functions:

1. It protects certain organs such as the brain, spinal cord, heart, and lungs.
2. It acts as a supportive framework for the body.
3. It acts as a system of levers, which the muscles can act on to stabilize and move the body.

1. Cranium
2. Clavicle
3. Sternum
4. Rib
5. Humerus
6. Radius
7. Ulna
8. Pubis
9. Carpus
10. Metacarpals

11. Phalanges
12. Femur
13. Patella
14. Tibia
15. Fibula
16. Tarsus
17. Metatarsals
18. Phalanges
19. Cervical vertebrae (7)

20. Scapula
21. Thoracic vertebrae (12)
22. Lumbar vertebrae (5)
23. Illium
24. Sacrum
25. Ischium

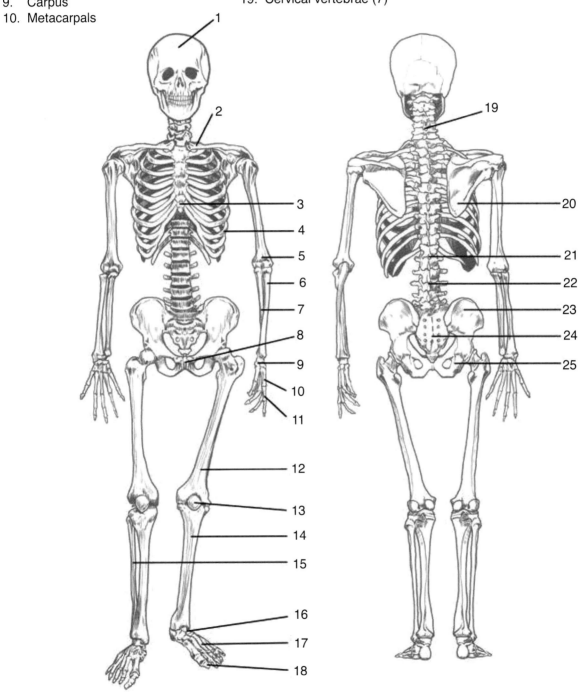

Figure 1.2 The passive (skeletal) system.

The bones of the skeleton are typically divided into two main groups: the axial skeleton and the appendicular skeleton. The adult axial skeleton is composed of approximately 80 bones that form the skull, spine, and rib cage. It provides the foundation for the body and protects the brain, spinal cord, and major organs.

The appendicular skeleton is composed of 126 bones that make up the scapula and upper limbs as well as the pelvis and the lower limbs. This collection of bones provides the primary lever systems that enable humans to exert force to move the trunk, its limbs, or any external objects.

Through biomechanical analysis and research on muscular action, any major movement of the trunk or limbs is initiated with either movement or stabilization of the spine. Therefore it is logical to assume that safe and efficient exercise technique should dedicate at least as much emphasis on the stabilization or movement responsibilities of the axial skeleton as it does for providing instruction on movement of the appendicular skeleton. Often resistance training technique focuses more on movement of the limbs and the weight while ignoring the importance of stabilizing spinal positioning and posture. The techniques presented in this book consider the role of the axial skeleton and the muscles that control it in an exercise movement. For easy reference, figure 1.2 on page 5 details the structure of the passive (skeletal) system.

Joints

Bones come together to form joints and are held together by connective tissues that are also vital components of the passive system. Each joint of the body is uniquely constructed to allow for movements in certain directions and ranges while also limiting movement in other directions. There are three general classifications of joints based on their amounts of articulation, or available movement: fibrous, cartilaginous, and synovial joints.

Fibrous joints allow for very little, if any, movement because of the small amount of space between bone endings. They include the joints of the skull, the joints between the radius and ulna of the lower arm, and the distal connection of the fibula and tibia of the lower leg.

Cartilaginous joints allow for some movement, but the movement is limited because of their proportionally higher compositions of collagen to elastin fiber, such as the joints that connect the ribs to the sternum. Both fibrous and cartilaginous joints have specific and important functions, although they do not provide for significant body movements.

Synovial joints account for most of the joints of the human body and vary on the amount of motion they provide. There are three types of synovial joints, which are categorized by the number of directions in which they can rotate around their given axis. They are uniaxial, biaxial, and multiaxial joints and are pictured in figures 1.3a, 1.3b, and 1.3c.

Uniaxial joints have only the direction of rotation and operate much like a hinge. The elbow and the phalangeal joints of the fingers are examples of uniaxial joints. Biaxial joints such as the wrist, ankle, and knee (when flexed) allow for movement in two perpendicular planes. Multiaxial joints, such as the shoulder and hip, allow for movement in all three planes of motion, so they provide the largest degrees and varieties of possible movement.

Connective Tissue

A joint's ability to move is determined in part by the structure and congruence of the bones themselves. Connective tissues are what hold the bones together and regulate the type, direction, and range of motion between the bone endings. Noncontractile, connective tissue contains high amounts of proprioceptors that relay vital information to the control system relevant to joint position, movement, and stress. This neural connection provides for the ability of the passive and control systems to interact directly. Two major types of passive connective tissues that assist with stabilization and regulation of joint movement are ligaments and joint capsules.

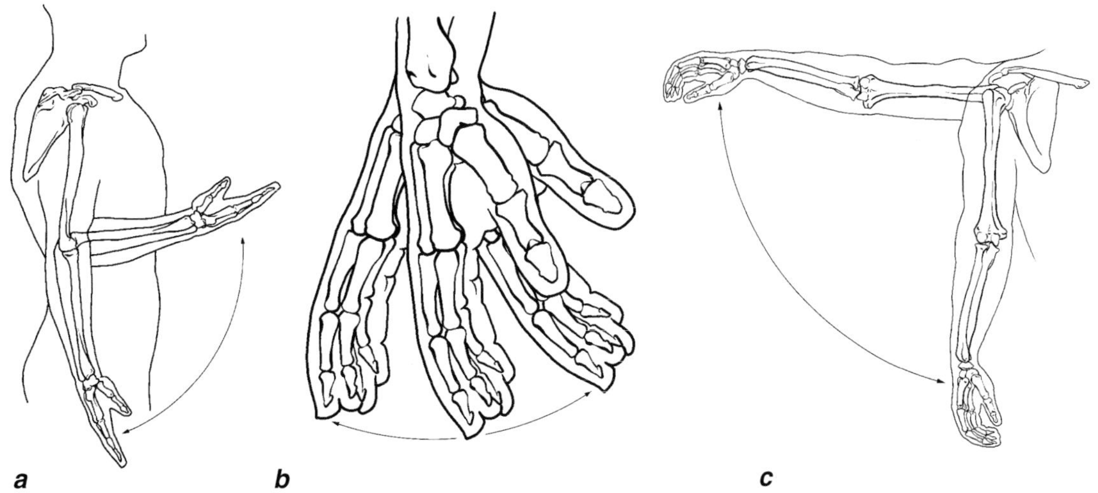

Figure 1.3 Examples of the three types of synovial joints: *(a)* uniaxial, *(b)* biaxial, and *(c)* multiaxial.

Ligaments connect bone to bone and consist primarily of strong collagen fibers arranged parallel to each other with only small amounts of elastic fiber. They are designed to restrict joint movement within specific directions and within specific ranges of motion. They are not capable of any significant stretching without deformation or tearing. Therefore they are at risk when movement is forced at a joint in directions or at ranges outside their genetically determined limits. Ligaments can be separate or a part of the joint capsule located outside or inside the capsule itself. Ligament placement and design are relative to the function of the joint and its needs for mobility and stability.

Joint capsules enclose the joint, creating a cavity that holds fluid in the joint and also assists in the transfer of forces from bone to bone. The capsule is typically composed of two or more layers of regular collagenous tissue that forms a sleeve around the joint. The parallel collagen fiber arrangements of each layer are typically laid down at different angles to the adjacent layers. This enables the capsule to allow for movement in certain directions and still strongly resist movement in other directions. Capsules assist with joint stability and are sensitive to overstretching, which can deform and tear the capsule.

Cartilage is another substance found at synovial joints that does not play a connective role but should also be considered when analyzing joint movement and joint forces. Cartilage can also be damaged as a result of excessive joint movement or through exposure to compressive, distractive, or shearing forces. Damage to cartilage is often permanent and can occur suddenly or gradually depending on the range, force, or repetition of joint motion.

Hyaline, or *articular cartilage,* is a smooth, slick protective covering over bone endings at synovial joints. This cartilage assists in ease of joint movement. Though articular cartilage is constructed to absorb some force and friction, excessive pressure, repetitive mechanical wear, or excessive movement can degenerate articular cartilage. Osteoarthritis can develop in joints where articular cartilage is worn. Once osteoarthritis begins, it often continues to deteriorate joint surfaces, causing inflammation, pain, and decreased joint function.

Fibrocartilage contains high concentrations of collagenous fibers and is specially designed for absorbing shock. It is a thick, rubber-like material found in the vertebral disks of the spine, menisci of the knee, the pubic symphysis of the pelvis, and at other joints in need of the extra cartilage support or padding between bone surfaces. Though resilient, fibrocartilage is also susceptible to thinning, tearing, folding, and rupturing under high levels of or frequent exposure to impact forces and friction. The body's natural replacement of fibrocartilage is limited, which can often leave the joint with little or no disk substance and painful, inefficient joint movement.

Active System

The active system is composed of the muscles and their associated tendons and fascia. Any joint movement requires more muscle action than just those directly responsible for the actual limb or body movement. Numerous other muscles work simultaneously in order to maintain center of gravity; stabilize the spine, pelvis, scapula, and assisting joints; or neutralize other muscle actions associated with the motion. In fact, more than 600 voluntary muscles may play various roles in an integrated manner in order to optimally produce certain desired movements. Figure 1.4 depicts most of the major muscles of the human muscular system. Any fitness professional should invest in a few good anatomy texts that further detail muscle topography and depict the actual origin and insertion points. Through close analysis of tendon attachment sites of the muscles, you can better understand how most every muscle is designed to be dominant in a general plane of movement yet also capable of functioning in all three planes in order to assist other muscles with joint movement and stability.

The muscles of the body are the powerhouses for all movement and serve as the primary link between the control and passive systems. In fact, the interdependent relationship of the active system and the passive system gives rise to additional terminology often used by other authors and will occasionally be referenced in this text. The musculoskeletal system can be viewed as an interdependent relationship and the combined functions of the passive and active systems; likewise, the neuromuscular system represents the interdependent relationship and combined functions of the control and active systems. Figures 1.5a and 1.5b depict these common references for better understanding.

Basic Muscle Structure

The unique physiological properties of muscle tissue enable it to respond to the commands sent from the control system and then immediately produce the appropriate pulling forces that are then applied to the levers of the passive system in order to position, stabilize, and move the body. Figure 1.6 on page 10 illustrates the physiological structure of a typical fusiform muscle–tendon unit for better understanding of muscle structure and function.

Muscles are anchored to the bone through strong fibrous cords known as tendons. Each muscle is wrapped in a protective sheath and held together by deep fascia called the epimysium. Internally, the muscle consists of bundles of muscle fibers called fasciculi that are also wrapped in a protective sheath called the perimysium. Inside the fasciculi are the muscle fibers that run the full length of the muscle from origin to insertion and range from a few inches to over three feet in length. Muscle fibers are also wrapped in their own a protective fascia called the endomysium. This deep fascia helps with force production and allows for smooth sliding of adjacent fibers as the muscle lengthens and shortens. Fascia also discourages the development of adhesions between the adjacent fibers that can limit muscle function and cause pain. Inside each muscle fiber are the myofibrils that contain the contractile protein filaments known as myosin and actin. This is where actual muscle contraction is possible.

Myofibrils are divided into smaller units known as sarcomeres (figure 1.7), which house the myosin and actin filaments. When a muscle is stimulated through a signal from its specific motor unit, the impulse initiates a series of chemical reactions involving calcium and ATP (adenosine triphosphate) that results in a mechanical pulling action of the actin filaments across the myosin. This sliding effect of the filaments pulls the Z lines of each sarcomere within the muscle fiber closer together, which therefore shortens (contracts) the entire muscle. A motor unit is a single motor neuron and all the muscle fibers it integrates. According to the all-or-nothing theory of muscle contraction, if a signal is strong enough to activate any motor unit, all fibers of that unit will contract with maximal force.

1. Platysma
2. Deltoid
3. Pectoralis major
4. Biceps brachii
5. Pronator teres
6. Flexor group
7. External oblique
8. Rectus abdominis
9. Adductors
10. Sartorius
11. Rectus femoris
12. Vastus medialis
13. Peroneus longus
14. Tibialis anterior
15. Coracobrachialis
16. Brachialis
17. Internal oblique
18. Brachioradialis
19. Flexor digitorum
    superficialis

20. Trapezius
21. Deltoid
22. Triceps brachii
23. Latissimus dorsi
24. Extensor group
25. Gluteus maximus
26. Iliotibial tract
27. Biceps femoris
28. Semitendinosus

29. Gastrocnemius
30. Splenius capitis
31. Levator scapula
32. Rhomboids
33. Infraspinatus
34. Teres minor
35. Teres major
36. Erector spinae
37. Serratus posterior inferior
38. Gluteus minimus
39. Gluteus medius (cut)
40. Piriformis
41. Semimembranosus
42. Plantaris
43. Popliteus
44. Soleus

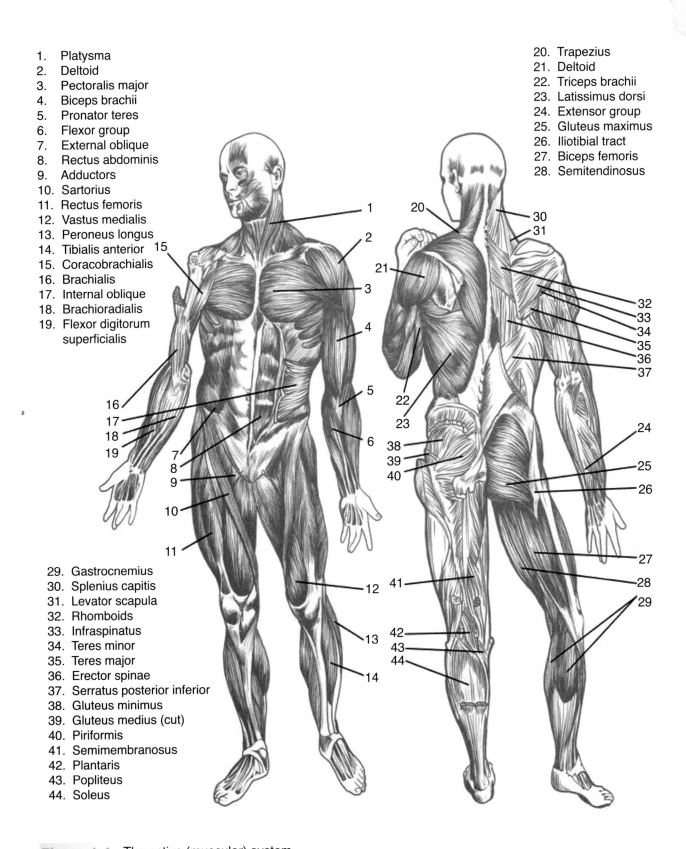

Figure 1.4 The active (muscular) system.

9

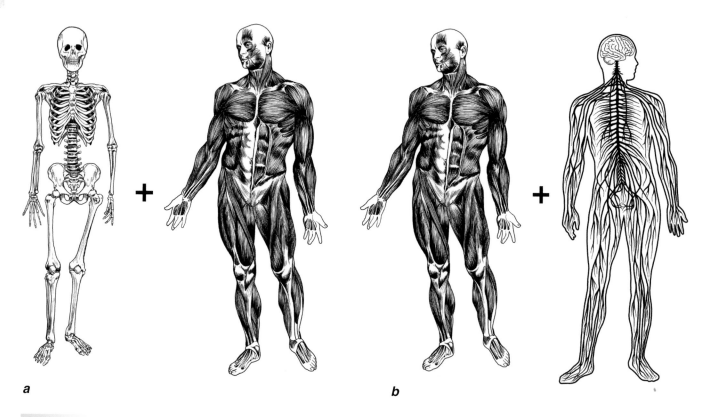

Figure 1.5 The (a) musculoskeletal system and (b) the neuromuscular system.

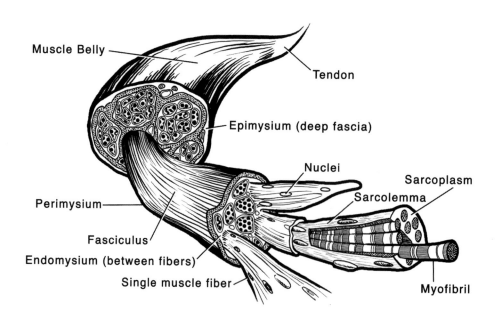

Figure 1.6 The muscle–tendon unit.

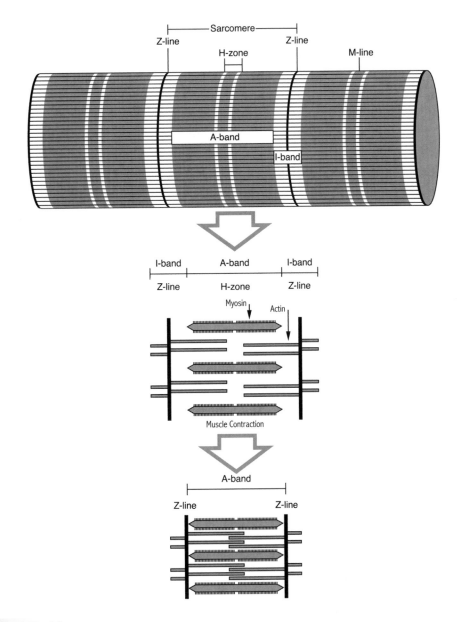

Figure 1.7 The sarcomere.

This simplified summary of neural and muscular interaction is the process in which muscles produce the varying levels of tension necessary for producing any type of muscle contraction. Muscles fulfill their various roles by providing different levels of force production through three types of muscular contractions.

- A concentric contraction is one in which the muscle–tendon unit produces ample force to create a joint movement and therefore shortens while contracting. The muscle would typically work as the agonist or the synergist with this type of contraction.
- An eccentric contraction occurs when the muscle–tendon unit produces just enough force to control its rate of lengthening. The muscle could be working as either the agonist (such as when lowering an object) or as the antagonist in order to decelerate limb or body movement.
- An isometric contraction is one in which the muscle–tendon unit neither shortens nor lengthens while still producing tension and a contractile force. Muscles would most often work as stabilizers or could perform a more quasi-isometric contraction and work as a neutralizer.

In addition to their active ability to contract, muscles have elastic properties that encourage them to return to their resting length once tension is removed. They also have plastic properties that resist being stretched too far. In fact, plastic properties of the muscle fascia can contribute to more than 40 percent of a joint's level of stiffness or flexibility. With proper stretching and active lengthening techniques, some of this resistance can be reduced through safe adaptations of the fascia. Consequently, repetitive inefficient stretching, ballistic stretching, or forced passive lengthening of a muscle can cause deformation of connective tissue, alter length–tension relationships, decrease muscle force production, and alter joint mechanics, all of which can lead to injury. For these reasons many experts now recommend active stretching over passive stretching. An active stretch is performed through direct use of an agonist muscle to lengthen the targeted antagonist. A passive stretch is accomplished through the means of an outside force such as gravity, another person, one's arms to pull on the limbs, or external anchors in order to stretch muscles. The differences, risks, and benefits associated with both passive and active stretching techniques are presented in chapter 3.

Muscles have the highest contractile force potential at or just slightly longer than resting length. Contractile force production is reduced when the muscle length is significantly shortened or lengthened before contraction. This is because the myosin and actin filaments have little room for additional cross-bridging when significantly shortened, or they are unable to begin optimal cross-bridging when significantly lengthened. Either scenario can drastically reduce muscle force output and is referred to as active insufficiency. Active insufficiency may be described as a muscle's diminished ability to produce active tension or force. The exercise techniques for each exercise in this book have been modified according to positioning and range of motion to account for all probable active insufficiency issues at each involved joint.

Actions and Roles of Muscles

Although muscles tend to dominate one plane of motion, they are designed to contribute in the other planes as well. The control system is designed to coordinate muscle synergies and recruit muscles for a variety of functions. Depending on the load, direction of resistance, and body position, muscles can function as agonists, antagonists, synergists, stabilizers, or neutralizers, though their roles may be subject to perception.

Agonists are muscles that act as the primary movers for performance of the desired motion. The agonists are responsible not only for accelerating the concentric movement but also for decelerating the eccentric movement. The agonists can also produce an isometric contraction to stabilize a set joint position. For example, the biceps muscle group during a biceps exercise accelerates elbow flexion, decelerates elbow extension, and also isometrically stabilizes the elbow at any point of the movement. In all three phases of this example, the biceps is still working as an agonist.

Antagonists are the muscles that work in direct opposition to the present movement. To contract any muscle, the antagonist muscle must release most of its tension. This action is known as reciprocal inhibition and is often depicted as a complete shutdown of the antagonist muscles during opposing movements. This view is oversimplified since muscle recruitment is affected by mechanoreceptors at the joint; complete antagonist inhibition is unlikely because it would alter joint mechanics. Antagonists play significant "braking" roles when performing fast concentric movements such as throwing a ball or swinging a golf club in order to decelerate the limb or trunk. All muscles work together harmoniously to produce joint motion and are never really antagonistic to each other.

Synergists are muscles that assist the agonists, or primary movers, with the movement. Their attachment angles and direction of pull are not as optimal for producing the movement as those muscles classified as the agonists but can still play important roles in joint motion and stabilization. The degree of assistance they offer depends on the amount of overall resistance, direction of resistance, and present capabilities of the agonists.

If the agonist is limited or inhibited because of either structural or neural issues, the synergist will often be forced to compensate. Chronic compensation can lead to synergistic dominance, which produces alterations in the relationship between muscle length and tension; decreases joint function; increases joint wear; and affects posture, gait, or performance of any gross movement pattern. Compensation and synergistic dominance affect the sensorimotor system as well as the skeletal and muscular systems, and may result in continued altered joint movement even if joint mechanics have been corrected.

Stabilizers are muscles that are used isometrically or quasi-isometrically to either hold a certain joint position or govern its movement. Muscles designed primarily for stabilization roles, such as the postural muscles of the spine and some of the deep core muscles, are referred to as tonic muscles. They are constructed for endurance and have low force output. However, most muscles designed for producing movement, known as phasic muscles, can also act as stabilizers when needed. Stabilization of certain joints is always a prerequisite in order to move others. This makes stabilization a critical role for muscles to perform and is why it is also considered an essential element of exercise technique.

Neutralizers are muscles that exert light forces to counteract an unwanted action of another muscle. For example, certain core muscles, such as the transverse abdominis and multifidi, work in concert with other core muscles to neutralize the shearing forces applied to the lumbar spine by the forward pull of the psoas and other hip flexors during gait movement. Without proper functioning of neutralizers, joint mechanics are altered and development of faulty motor patterns can cause compensation and an increased incidence of injury or joint degeneration.

Muscular Subsystems

Isolated joint movements may constitute a portion of a resistance training routine that addresses specific training needs or accomplishes certain goals. However, isolated joint or muscle actions are rarely performed in real life. Therefore, the control system rarely recruits individual muscles but rather recruits a concert of muscle synergies that work to stabilize, neutralize, accelerate, and decelerate the body as it moves. It is logical to deduce that a well-designed exercise program for most people should also be dominated by exercises that use multiple joint motions to produce general movement patterns and target muscle synergies as opposed to individual muscles. This should help to ensure that exercise programs offer benefits that transfer better to meeting the demands of life and sports. Isolated joint motion exercises can then be added to further develop specific musculature for aesthetic or performance-related goals.

Any repetitive movement pattern you perform often and consistently enough would feasibly recruit specific muscle synergies and develop improved intermuscular coordination. Muscle synergies are biomechanically linked subsystems that improve innate neurological relationships or develop new ones in order to produce more unique movement patterns. Once these neurological relationships are developed and reinforced, an imprint of the motor program is stored that allows for quick recall and recruitment of the muscle synergies developed to produce the specific desired movement pattern. There are five such muscle synergies, or subsystems, of the active muscular system that are highly involved in many common movements such as squatting, pushing, pulling, and walking. These subsystems have also been recognized for their critical roles in trunk and pelvis stabilization and control:

1. Inner unit (core)
2. Deep longitudinal subsystem (DLS)
3. Lateral subsystem (LS)
4. Posterior oblique subsystem (POS)
5. Anterior oblique subsystem (AOS)

Chapter 5, Resistance Exercise Selection, provides a summary of these subsystems and their associated roles for movement and stabilization of the body. You will also notice many exercises in chapters 7, 8, 9, 10, and 11 that identify these subsystems' involvement for the specific resisted movement.

Control System

The complexity of the design and inner workings of the entire control (sensorimotor) system (figure 1.8) is far beyond the scope of this book. Rather, we present the components of the control system and summarize their associated functions relative to performance of movement. This information will help you as a professional trainer, strength coach, or instructor to better understand the important factors necessary for efficient exercise selection and instruction of optimal technique, and it will empower you to design more effective exercise programs.

The control system, or sensorimotor system, is viewed as the central nervous system (CNS), peripheral sensory and motor nervous systems, and all sensory receptors that assist with providing information and feedback to the CNS. Humans receive continuous sensory information about the present environment through a number of sensory channels. The three primary sources for sensory information are visual input, vestibular input, and proprioception, which can be summed up as afferent input from peripheral sensory receptors and joint–muscle mechanoreceptors.

During any movement, visual and vestibular receptors sense changes in center of gravity and play an important role in body positioning and balance. Sensory receptors in the skin and cutaneous tissues sense changes in pressure and movement of soft tissue. Mechanoreceptors located in the muscles, joints, and connective tissues give continuous information and feedback on joint position, joint stability, joint movement, muscle length, muscle tension, and pressure from external and internal forces.

All this afferent information is routed to three different yet interactive areas of motor control depending on the complexity of the information and the familiarity of the various stimuli. Reflex actions and motor responses are then formulated to produce the desired movement. The three areas of motor control are as follows:

1. The spinal cord is responsible for managing immediate and automated reflex actions.

2. The lower brain organizes more complex responses and assists the higher brain in monitoring and modifying movement patterns.

3. The cerebral cortex is the higher brain, which is responsible for controlling the most complex responses, initiation of all voluntary movement, and storage of motor programs.

Each of these general areas of motor control will be summarized so that you can better understand where and how specific sensory information is processed in order to provide necessary data and feedback critical for specific motor responses and creation of movement patterns. Figure 1.9 depicts the brain and origin of the spinal cord for a visual reference of the various sections of the primary control center of the sensorimotor system and the three general areas of motor control.

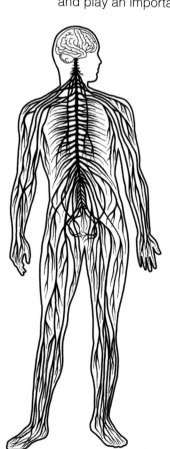

Figure 1.8 The control system.

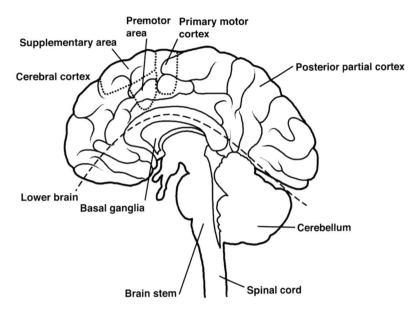

Figure 1.9 Motor control areas of the brain.

Spinal Cord

The spinal cord is made up of two-way tracks of nerve fibers. It carries both sensory fibers and motor fibers between the periphery organs and brain. It allows for the continuous flow of afferent information from the sensory receptors to the higher levels of motor control. It also contains the efferent motor fibers carrying command information from the cerebrum to the periphery organs or muscles.

One branch of the sensory nerves terminates in the gray matter of the spinal cord while another branch is carried to the higher levels of control in the brain. This enables the spinal cord to react autonomously to certain stimuli without processing or commands from a higher level of control. These reflex actions, such as pulling the hand away from a hot stove or quickly regaining balance after a near fall, are critical for protection of the body and are also involved in development of neuromuscular coordination.

Some reflex actions, such as those involved in control of center of gravity or maintenance of balance, can be enhanced through repeated exposure to the stimuli or exercise. However, because sensory input is highly specific and inclusive of all environmental factors, so are the associated reflex actions. Therefore training adaptations made while training within a specific environment or with a specific tool most likely will not transfer well when performing similar movements in a different environment or when using a different tool.

Motor commands are sent through the spinal cord with two types of anterior motor neurons: alpha neurons and gamma neurons. Alpha motor neurons are larger motor neurons that innervate the large skeletal muscles of the body. Alpha motor neurons can innervate a small amount of fibers for fine control such as for the fingers and toes. Yet, they can also innervate up to several hundred muscle fibers in larger muscles for gross control of major joint movements. The spinal cord along with the brain regulates the excitation or recruitment of motor units based on sensory information and the perceived need.

Gamma motor neurons innervate small intrafusal fibers and mechanoreceptors within the joints and skeletal muscle. There are two classes of gamma motor neurons. One type controls dynamic sensitivity or movement, and the other controls static sensitivity or stabilization. These specialized motor neurons are constantly influenced by information provided by the joint mechanoreceptors, such as the Ruffini endings, Pacinian corpuscles, Golgi-Mazzoni endings, and ligament endings, as well as the information sent forth from the muscle spindles and Golgi tendon organs (GTOs). Gamma motor neurons play a critical role in both dynamic and static stabilization of the joint as well as the production of joint movement through the triggering of associated alpha motor neurons and recruitment of various muscle synergies.

Muscle spindles are located in the belly of the muscle. They monitor length of muscle or rate of change in length. Muscle spindles are extremely sensitive to the lengthening of a muscle and have both dynamic and static stretch reflexes. When activated, they can immediately signal the recruitment of motor units to create increased tension in a muscle in order to slow down the speed of lengthening or attempt to completely halt joint movement in order to protect the muscle or joint from harm. Although this stretch reflex action is believed to be a protective mechanism, it may also be manipulated and used to produce plyometric actions of the muscle. The stretch reflex produces an elastic recoil of the muscle–tendon unit to increase force potential for jumping movements and throwing activities. However, muscle damage can also result from an untimely stretch reflex or muscle-spindle activation. This can occur when the neuromuscular system is unprepared for the quick and forceful muscular lengthening associated with a sudden body or limb movement.

Golgi tendon organs (GTOs) are another type of mechanoreceptor and are located in the tendon. They monitor muscle tension and its rate of change as opposed to changes in length. GTOs immediately transmit information to the CNS relating to the degrees of tension on the tendons and muscles throughout the body. When tension is too high or increased too quickly within a muscle, the GTOs send an immediate alarm that can trigger a partial or complete inhibition within that muscle. This also appears to be a protective mechanism to preserve muscle and tendon structures. There is a dampening effect of both GTO and muscle spindle activity when exposed to the stimuli gradually or often enough so that the entire system becomes conditioned to the speed and relative tensions associated with the movement. This provides a sound rationale for regular practice of the specific movements that a person wants to improve. Also a specific movement pattern warm-up with gradual progressions in range and speed of movement as well as gradual applications of any resistance would be logical to perform before attempting any movement at full power.

It is clear that there is a difference in the mechanoreceptor activity and motor unit recruitment required for stabilization of a joint versus movement of a joint. Therefore, you can conclude that almost every joint and its associated musculature should be trained to provide both stabilization and optimal movement, each of which will require different training stimuli to accomplish. This is the reason that there is just as much, if not more, emphasis placed on stabilization during any exercise presented in this book as there is on producing movement. The stabilization of the specific positioning and the posture options are stressed as critical elements of technique for every resistance exercise presented and perhaps offer more benefits than the exercise movement itself.

Lower Brain

The lower brain consists of the brain stem, basal ganglia, and cerebellum. Several descending pathways of motor control are directly or indirectly under the control of the lower brain. Certain afferent sensory information is processed at this level along with efferent commands in order to modify a movement for greater efficiency.

The brain stem is the stalk of the brain connecting it to the spinal cord. All sensory and motor information must pass through it. It contains a specialized collection of neurons that coordinate skeletal muscle function and modify specific control functions of the body. The brain stem also plays a significant role in stability training and in maintaining balance over a base of support.

The cerebellum is the ultimate modifier. It assists the primary motor cortex and the basal ganglia to adjust the actual movement patterns being produced to conform to the desired motor patterns established by the higher brain. The cerebellum processes relayed decisions for desired movements developed in the motor cortex and compares these commands with the sensory feedback from the various receptors. It then evaluates and attempts to modify actual movements by eliminating inefficient responses or correcting delays to motor commands, or it compensates for sudden changes in external stimuli or loss of internal control. The cerebellum is always attempting to learn how to best perform a movement based on all available information and is also highly involved in ballistic movements such as running, jumping, and agility training.

The basal ganglia is much like the assistant manager to the higher brain. Its primary role is to assist with the control of complex motor activities. Almost all sensory and motor nerve fibers connecting the cerebral cortex with the spinal cord pass between the basal ganglia. Various nuclei are contained in the basal ganglia that assist the cerebral cortex with specific functions. One of these nuclei is the caudate nucleus, which plays an important role in cognitive control of difficult or new movement patterns. However, another unique responsibility delegated to the basal ganglia is to initiate and control repetitive and continuous movement patterns such as walking and running, which require far less conscious thought and are more autonomous movements.

Cerebral Cortex

The cerebral cortex, or higher brain, is the general manager of the sensorimotor system responsible for control of the most complex motor patterns and initiation of all voluntary movements. It is composed of the upper and most outer areas of the brain consisting of two hemispheres connected by the corpus callosum. It also has two functional areas concerned with movement: the anterior motor cortex and the posterior somatic sensory cortex. The cerebral cortex simultaneously processes input gathered in the somatic sensory cortex while controlling the different functions of the motor cortex and coordinating the various activities of the lower brain and spinal cord. Desired motor commands developed within the cerebral cortex are then sent to the lower centers of the control system for further development and modification. Final movement commands and stabilization strategies are then passed along to the active muscle system for final execution.

The anterior motor cortex can be further divided into three smaller areas that perform specific functions. The primary motor cortex controls fine voluntary movements. Its right side controls the left side of the body and its left side controls the right side of the body. It is responsible for consciously controlled skilled movements and works directly with the spinal cord through the corticospinal tract for control and integration of reflex actions.

The premotor area of the motor cortex is involved in the development of finely skilled movement. It works with the primary motor cortex, the basal ganglia, and the thalamus to form a system for efficient coordinated muscle activity. The supplementary area functions synergistically with the premotor area to help with postural adjustments and is highly involved in bilateral movements of the body. As normal gait patterns and most other functional movements performed in life or sports involve contralateral movements of the legs and arms, bilateral limb movement is not common. However, in the gym bilateral limb movements such as barbell pressing, dumbbell or cable bicep and tricep exercises, squats, and leg presses often dominate many people's programs.

Neuromuscular Efficiency and Motor Learning

The combination of the control system and the active system (neuromuscular system) can become more synchronized for performing a specific complex movement or an exercise through repeated practice as neuromuscular efficiency is developed. This means the movement can be performed more skillfully with less conscious effort and with less metabolic cost. Efficient movement involves both intermuscular and intramuscular coordination.

Intermuscular coordination is the ability of the neuromuscular system to orchestrate the most efficient recruitment of agonists, synergists, stabilizers, and neutralizers for a given movement. Intramuscular coordination is the ability of the neuromuscular system to control specific recruitment of motor units and muscle fibers within the same muscle. This process involves number encoding, pattern encoding, and rate encoding. Number encoding is basically the total number of muscle fibers recruited. Pattern encoding deals more with the synchronization of the appropriate types of muscle fibers recruited. Rate encoding is the rate at which muscle fiber is recruited or activated.

Neuromuscular efficiency can be described as the ability of the neuromuscular system to learn, store, recall, perform, and modify desired motor programs. Neuromuscular efficiency requires quick processing of all afferent sensory information with simultaneous coordination of efferent motor commands complete with the required intermuscular and intramuscular coordination and stabilization strategies necessary for meeting environmental demands. High levels of neuromuscular efficiency also demand advanced levels of innate kinesthesia, which is the awareness of body positioning and joint movement relative to space. A person's agility and athletic ability are also tied closely to levels of neuromuscular efficiency.

Improving neuromuscular efficiency and coordination is a process. The related systems for improved intermuscular and intramuscular control; integration of reflex actions; improved motor responses; and the learning, refining, and modifying of motor programs all take time and repeated exposure to the specific stimuli. Coordination can be classified into three basic stages that relate to the level of present motor control: general coordination, special coordination, and specific coordination.

General Coordination: Cognitive Control   This stage is characterized by the need for cognitive, or conscious, control of voluntary movement. The person must think through the movement as it is being performed and rely heavily on visual and vestibular input because proprioception information is too new and unfamiliar at this stage.

Special Coordination: Associated Control   At this stage the person has become more comfortable and begins to feel the proper movement patterns. The person relies less on visual and auditory information and makes more use of proprioception. The person installs stabilization and balance strategies and also begins to use feedback information to refine the skill and discard undesired motion.

Specific Coordination: Autonomous Control   This stage is the highest level of motor control. It is characterized by the performance of the skill through stored motor programs with no conscious thought. The neuromuscular system carries on with automatic reflex actions and response commands to all environmental variables, and the movement pattern is free of all superfluous motion.

General Movement Patterns

There is an infinite number of possible motor programs that could be produced by the human body, which prompts the question of how the brain can possibly learn, store, and recall such large amounts of finely detailed data. In answer to this question, Schmidt and Wrisberg, in their book *Motor Learning and Performance,* present the concept of generalized motor programs. This theory proposes that general motor patterns, as opposed to specific detailed movements, are stored in the higher levels of the brain for quick recall when needed. Then, depending on the afferent information from the various receptors, these general motor programs can then be quickly modified at the appropriate level to meet the environmental demands. This storage and recall process is deemed to be most efficient for production and modification of optimal movement. More detailed information on the development and continued use of general movement patterns and how general movement patterns relate to exercise selection, exercise technique, and exercise program design are covered in the following chapters.

Joint Mechanics

As presented in chapter 1, any movement of the body, no matter how complex or simple, requires the interdependent actions of the control, active, and passive systems. Even the smallest of isolated joint motions will necessitate the integrated work of hundreds of timed muscle contractions in order to stabilize the body and limbs and neutralize unwanted simultaneous motion while accelerating and decelerating the actual joint motion.

The typical presentation of anatomical movement, which depicts only isolated concentric joint motions performed against an imagined all-encompassing resistance (if the body were moving inside a tank of water floating in space), is not an accurate representation of how muscles and joints function when moving naturally in the presence of gravity. It is also important to consider the fact that the body rarely performs isolated joint movements in everyday movement other than when done intentionally as a part of an exercise program to accomplish specific training goals. For these reasons, the traditional study of kinesiology has limited applications to how the body actually performs functional movement. However, it is important for you as a fitness professional to be able to link all individual joint motions with the specific muscles most directly responsible for concentric action or acceleration of the movement. Only then can you begin to recognize the muscles' eccentric actions that provide for deceleration and their isometric or quasi-isometric actions needed for functional movement and stabilization.

This chapter is provided as a study guide and a quick reference for learning basic isolated joint and muscle mechanics. Keep in mind that even though joints may appear to move in only one plane, they most often make minute shifts and movements in all three planes simultaneously. Likewise, though many muscles are aligned to operate dominantly in one plane, most muscles are capable of assisting with movement at some level in all three planes of motion. You can see this fact by cross-referencing the lists of muscle actions and noting their involvement in other joint motions in different planes.

Movements are presented in a traditional three-plane format as pictured in figure 2.1 and incorporate the following premises:

- Joint movement begins from a preset anatomical standing position.
- Each joint movement is considered in isolation and performed in only one general plane of motion.
- It is assumed that all listed joint motions are the result of active concentric muscle actions against a directly opposing force.
- Only the muscles most directly involved with the specific movement of that joint are listed.
- The terminology of joint motion may not be consistent with the terminology used in other sources.

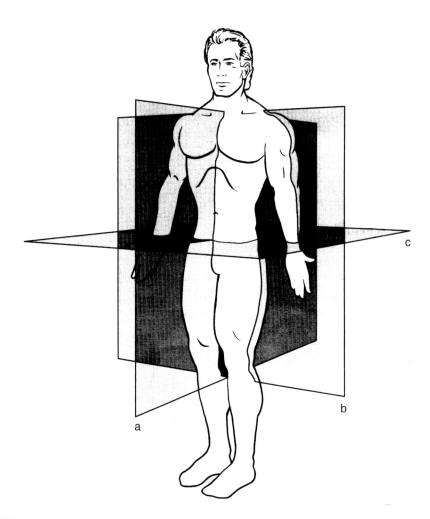

Figure 2.1 The planes of motion: *(a)* the median plane, *(b)* the frontal plane, and *(c)* the horizontal plane.

Joint Motions of the Median Plane

The median plane is also known as the sagittal plane. It divides the body down the middle into left and right halves. Most human movement takes place in the median plane. The joint motions of flexion and extension are the primary movements of the median plane and occur at the ankle, knee, hip, spine, shoulder, elbow, and wrist. Scapular protraction and retraction are also considered movements of the median plane.

Ankle Flexion (Dorsiflexion)
Tibialis anterior
Extensor hallucis longus
Extensor digitorum longus
Peroneus tertius

Ankle Extension (Plantar Flexion)
Peroneus longus
Peroneus brevis
Triceps surae
Flexor hallucis longus
Tibialis posterior
Flexor digitorum longus

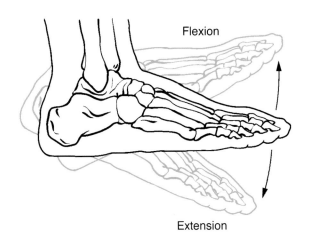

Knee Flexion
Biceps femoris (long and short heads)
Semitendinosus
Semimembranosus
Popliteus
Gastrocnemius
Sartorius
Gracilis

Knee Extension
Vastus lateralis
Vastus medialis
Vastus intermedius
Rectus femoris
Tensor fasciae latae
Gluteus maximus (superficial portion)

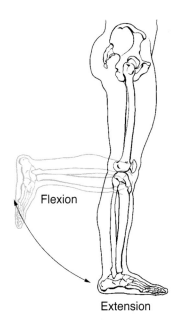

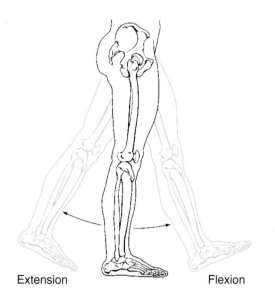

Extension   Flexion

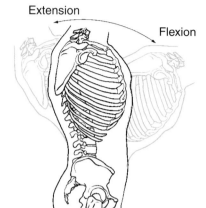

Extension   Flexion

Hip Flexion

Psoas
Iliacus
Rectus femoris
Tensor fasciae latae
Gluteus minimus and medius
(anterior portions)
Sartorius
Pectineus
Gracilis

Hip Extension

Gluteus maximus
Biceps femoris (long head)
Semimembranosus
Semitendinosus
Gluteus medius
(posterior portion)
Adductor magnus

Trunk Flexion

Rectus abdominis
External obliques
Internal obliques

Trunk Extension

Spinalis group
Longissimus group
Iliocostalis group
Transversospinalis group
Interspinalis
Intertransversarri

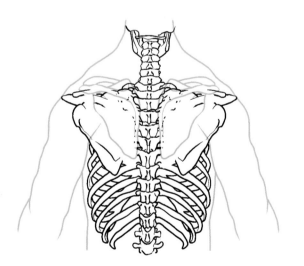

Retraction

Scapular Retraction (Adduction)

Mid trapezius
Rhomboids
Lower trapezius
Upper trapezius

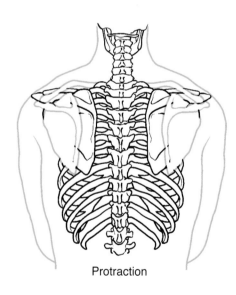

Protraction

Scapular Protraction (Abduction)

Mid serratus anterior
Upper serratus anterior (superior)
Lower serratus anterior (inferior)

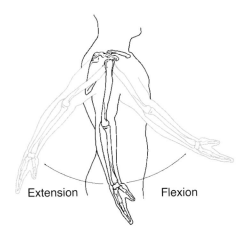

Extension | Flexion

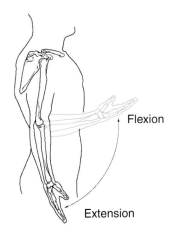

Flexion

Extension

Shoulder Flexion

Anterior deltoid
Pectoralis major
Coracobrachialis

Shoulder Extension

Latissimus dorsi
Posterior deltoid
Teres minor

Elbow Flexion

Biceps brachii
Brachioradialis
Brachialis

Elbow Extension

Triceps (long head)
Triceps (lateral head)
Triceps medial head
(deep head)
Anconeus

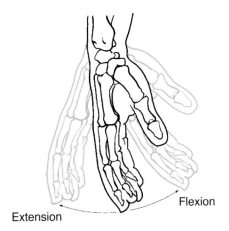

Extension | Flexion

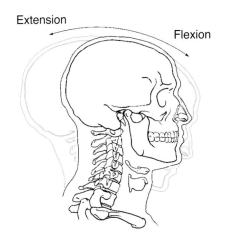

Extension | Flexion

Wrist Flexion

Flexor carpi radialis
Palmaris longus
Flexor carpi ulnaris

Wrist Extension

Extensor carpi radialis
longus
Extensor carpi radialis brevis
Extensor carpi ulnaris

Neck Flexion

Longus colli
Longus capitis
Rectus capitis anterior
Sternocleidomastoid
Anterior scalene
Mid scalene
Suprahyoid group
(accessory)
Infrahyoid group (accessory)

Neck Extension

Splenius cervicis
Splenius capitis
Semispinalis cervicis
Semispinalis capitis
Spinalis capitis
Longissimus cervicis
Longissimus capitis
Rectus capitis posterior
major
Rectus capitis posterior
minor
Levator scapulae
Trapezius

Joint Motions of the Frontal Plane

The frontal plane, sometimes referred to as the coronal plane, divides the body through the side into front and back halves. Joint movements of abduction and adduction of the wrist, shoulder, and hip, as well as inversion and eversion of the ankle, scapular elevation, depression, upward rotation, downward rotation, and trunk lateral flexion of the spine, are all movements of the frontal plane.

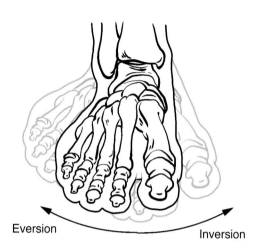

Eversion   Inversion

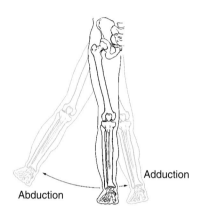

Adduction

Abduction

**Ankle Eversion
(Partial Pronation)**

Peroneus longus

Peroneus brevis

Peroneus tertius

Extensor digitorum longus
(lateral portion)

**Ankle Inversion
(Partial Supination)**

Extensor hallucis longus

Tibialis anterior

Tibialis posterior

Flexor digitorum longus

Flexor hallucis longus

Triceps surae

Hip Abduction

Gluteus medius

Gluteus minimus

Tensor fasciae latae

Gluteus maximus
(superficial portion)

Piriformis

Obturators

Gemelli

Sartorius

Hip Adduction

Adductor magnus

Adductor longus

Adductor brevis

Pectineus

Gracilis

Psoas

Iliacus

Trunk Lateral Flexion

Internal oblique (ipsilateral)

Quadratus lumborum (ipsilateral)

Rectus abdominis (ipsilateral)

Erector spinae (ipsilateral)

Latissimus dorsi (ipsilateral)

Transversospinalis group (ipsilateral)

Intertransversari (ipsilateral)

Flexion

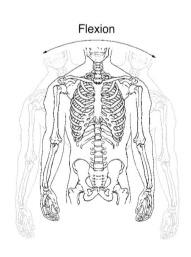

Strength and Tempo

Because strength increases are related to neurological adaptations, specific types of strength can be developed through different training techniques, particularly when implementing changes in the speed of movement. Tempo assignments can elicit significantly different strength adaptations and are necessary for targeting some of the different types of strength gains that may be desired. For example, a tempo assignment that promotes a longer pause at the eccentric isometric phase of each repetition would be ideal for developing static strength or starting strength, depending on the prescribed tempo of the other three phases of each repetition. On the other hand, working with a faster eccentric movement followed by a quick ballistic concentric movement with no pause at the eccentric isometric phase would incorporate a stretch reflex of the muscle as part of the technique. This would be consistent with the desire to increase explosive strength and power for that general movement pattern. More information related to tempo is in chapter 4, which should help you decide the proper speed and changes to speed of movement that would elicit the desired strength adaptations.

Endurance

Endurance is often thought to be solely an adaptation of the cardiorespiratory systems and associated primarily with increases of maximal oxygen consumption ($\dot{V}O_2$max). This misconception has led to training protocols for endurance athletes that dramatically overlook or completely ignore the possible benefits of strength training. The development of increased local muscular endurance that can be attained through resistance training is valuable for improved performance in endurance activities. Some level of strength is always involved in any event because there is no movement on this planet that is a nonresisted movement.

Local muscular endurance is the ability of the muscle to maintain the optimal force production necessary for the movement for an extended period. Local muscular endurance is derived from the development of endurance strength. The more strength required for the movement, the larger part endurance strength plays in its contribution to the endurance activity. For example, research on mastery-level middle-distance runners showed that a decrease in performance was associated primarily with local muscular fatigue, which leads to compensational movement patterns and a decrease in stride length as opposed to decreases in stride frequency. In other words, the decreased performance was due more to a loss of muscular endurance strength rather than a loss of cardiorespiratory endurance.

Further research comparing $\dot{V}O_2$max levels of top endurance athletes has shown very little correlation with performance. This proves that other contributing factors are associated with optimal performance in any endurance event that needs to be trained, apart from conditioning the cardiorespiratory system and increasing $\dot{V}O_2$max. Any movement performed for endurance will require the use of specific muscle synergies. Therefore, endurance is also dependent on specialized adaptations of certain skeletal muscles, particularly in regard to their level of endurance strength. Improvements in intramuscular control, such as the number, pattern, and rate encoding of muscle fibers, are also a key to improved endurance.

Conditioning programs for improved endurance should prepare the muscles for the onset of blood lactate accumulation (OBLA), which is the beginning of anaerobic threshold. This is when the anaerobic processes of ATP production for muscle contraction begin to become prominently involved, which decreases aerobic processes and limits endurance. Training should aim to develop lactic acid tolerance, which is the ability to continue adequate motor unit recruitment in the presence of higher blood lactate levels and reduced pH. Training should also strive to work the muscles to actually use lactic acid more efficiently as an intermediate energy source, thereby delaying OBLA while continuing to perform optimally. Resistance training circuits incorporating loading techniques such as supersets and drop sets as well as interval training can improve endurance strength of the specific muscles targeted and increase overall endurance.

Resistance training has been shown to increase a person's ability to obtain better gains in hemoglobin content and myoglobin content than straight aerobic training can provide. These are significant findings because increased hemoglobin and myoglobin are critical for improved endurance. This again demonstrates the potential benefits of adding specialized resistance training programs to any endurance athlete's training regimen to improve overall performance.

Endurance is not just a result of an isolated metabolic process; it relies heavily on neurological adaptations as well. Many endurance activities require the predominant use of repetitive movement patterns. This also requires specific repetitive joint movements and muscle actions to efficiently reproduce the movement pattern for prolonged periods. More specifically, mechanoreceptor activity within each involved joint and muscle will also have to adapt to specific conditions relative to joint angles of motion, joint range of motion, joint speed of motion, and joint force production and reductions associated with the overall movement pattern. This is necessary for coordinating motor unit encoding and muscle fiber recruitment for management of all related reflex actions and motor commands in response to feedback and environmental changes. Any breakdowns in these neural processes of the control and active systems will immediately tax the musculoskeletal system and result in decreased endurance.

Any reflex actions needed for the event and all voluntary movement will need to become less cognitively controlled and more automated for greater efficiency and improved metabolic conservation. Stabilization strategies will also need to become more easily managed with possible backup strategies prepared, as fatigue begins and compensation becomes more prevalent. It is probable that effective compensation patterns of movement will also need to be developed by the control system when preparing for competition in extreme endurance events such as marathons and triathlons. Even with training it is likely that all involved agonists and synergists will have different fatigue levels.

Changes in environmental factors such as temperature, terrain, elements, and specific equipment can also affect endurance and induce compensation strategies in order to continue performance in unfamiliar conditions. Compensation always has definite ramifications on the programming of the neuromuscular system and places increased stress and wear on the musculoskeletal system. However, compensation is a necessary action of the body for continued movement after joint actions are altered or as fatigue occurs, and it often begins to decrease endurance and performance far before it is visibly noticeable. For these reasons, endurance training should include as many as possible of the potential variables that may be encountered in life or sport situations for optimal adaptation to occur.

Stability

Stability, or stabilization for our purposes, is the internal ability to control all desired movement or nonmovement of the body and its segments in response to all internal and external forces and changes in center of gravity. Adopting this definition means that stabilization may be a static demand, a dynamic demand, or a balance demand, with most movements requiring a combined blend of all three. Even a simple walk around the block would require certain amounts of dynamic stability with some contributions of static stability, and it may even require minor levels of balance depending on the terrain and abilities of the person. Stability for any movement relies on specific types of strength and will also require some level of balance; it can also be influenced by joint mobility factors and even endurance factors.

Static Stability

Static stability is characterized by the joint's demonstration of the ability to hold a specific position. Static stability is accomplished through primarily isometric actions and is dependent on the present static strength of all involved muscles. The joint may be completely motionless, or it may be moving in space. For example, you may observe the static stability of the spine while it is completely motionless during a dumbbell biceps curl, or you may witness it during a squat movement in which the spine is again held stable yet is allowed to move in space. Both require varying levels of isometric contraction of the trunk muscles where the muscles are neither lengthening nor shortening yet are producing appropriate levels of force to provide for static stability.

Dynamic Stability

Dynamic stability can be considered centrification, which is characterized by the ability to control the joint axis to allow for joint motion within a specific range or within a selected plane. For example, both the hips and ankles are directly involved in median-plane flexion and extension during a narrow-stance squat movement. However, they must still be dynamically stabilized from moving into unwanted pronation or supination through the horizontal and frontal planes. Dynamic stability is often the result of combined controlled dynamic, isometric, and quasi-isometric muscle actions. Dynamic stability is also required when stability is needed on quick demand to support the joints during a sudden-impact force. This can be viewed as impact stability and is critical for any sports that involve jumping, quick changes of direction, bracing for an external force, or even just walking.

Stability requires the interaction of all three of the major systems also used for movement. The passive (skeletal) system, apart from its unique structural design and its own connective tissues, relies heavily on the force productions and reductions generated within the active (muscular) system for stabilization. This system in turn receives all reflex actions and motor commands from the control (sensorimotor) system. Therefore, stability is not just a product but rather a continuing process during any movement that is limited by the weakness or breakdown of any one of these systems. For example, if the control system fails to supply the proper reflex or command quickly enough, stability is compromised or lost. If, on the other hand, the active system receives the command but lacks the muscular strength, reaction, or endurance, stability is again compromised or lost. In either case, the passive system can be viewed as the last resort for stabilization. Any breakdown of stability here results in a total or partial collapse with a high probability for deformation or injury of the joint and possibly to other areas of the body as well. This provides a strong rationale for some level of stability and balance training in most everyone's program despite perception of overall goals. More specific information on stabilization training is presented in chapter 4.

Balance

Balance is an intricate part of stability. It is the process of maintaining center of gravity within the body's base of support. Balance relies predominantly on the activation of specialized reflex actions that vary from small shifting responses of the ankle or hip to stepping strategies and associated upper-extremity movement to regain center of gravity.

Balance reflexes can be divided into two major classifications: body-righting reflexes and tilting-response reflexes. Many sport and life movements may require a specific blend of both reflex actions, but most activities can be considered as a dominant demand of one over the other. Figures 3.2 and 3.3 depict the two major types of balance challenges.

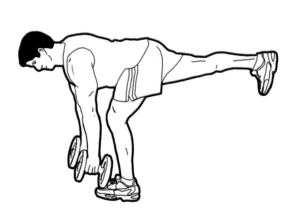

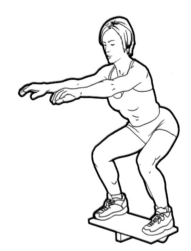

Figure 3.2 Body-righting reflex challenge.

Figure 3.3 Tilting-response reflex challenge.

Body-righting reflexes tend to dominate when a person stands or moves on a stable surface, such as when performing a dumbbell reverse lunge off a stable step or when a gymnast performs her routine on a balance beam. Tilting-response reflexes tend to dominate when moving across or standing on a supporting surface that is itself unstable or tends to shift or move.

Choosing the appropriate balance challenge is essential in order to train and improve the desired reflex action of the neuromuscular system as the different types of balance reflex adaptions do not transfer well if at all. It is also important to remember that any balance and stabilization strategies need to be programmed, a certain volume of exposure to the stimulus is required. In other words, it must be practiced often enough for the neuromuscular system to make the adaptation necessary for improved ability.

Mobility

At the other end of the same spectrum of joint stability is joint mobility. The integrity of every joint is dependent on both abilities; optimal performance has the ideal ratio of stability to mobility for all involved joints. Some movements or activities may require greater ranges of motion, while others would benefit from more stability and less available motion. Mobility is related to the joint's possible range of motion (ROM), which is difficult to determine since ROM varies under different conditions.

Technically, mobility is not synonymous with flexibility. Oddly enough, flexibility is often defined as all soft tissues' level of extensibility, which is related to its allowance for joint motion. In some kinesiology texts, flexibility is also used only to describe the degree of motion within the median plane and is specific to only the joint motion of flexion, such as when moving the arm forward. Therefore the degree to which you can move the arm backward would be termed *extensibility*, and how far you can move it out to the side would be *abductability*, and so forth. In this text we use the word *mobility* to describe the degree of joint motion regardless of plane or specific joint actions.

Two basic types of mobility are typically presented: passive and active mobility. Passive mobility refers to joint ROM produced when the muscles are inactive and a force outside that joint is responsible for limb or body movement. Active mobility is the degree of joint motion produced from forces generated inside the body through voluntary or reflex actions of the muscles.

Research has shown that there can be large degrees of difference between measurements of passive ROM and active ROM in many people, which has been termed the *flexibility deficit*.

This demonstrates that increases in passive ROM do not necessarily increase active ROM. Many experts believe that one's flexibility deficit is proportional to one's possible risk of injury because passive ROM without muscle control places the joint in a position of instability and risk. Some, however, believe that passive ROM beyond active ROM can be beneficial because it may function as a protective reserve in situations where a sudden force takes the joint past its normal operating limit. However, research supporting this concept is not available and the theory is highly questionable.

The type, exact direction, speed, and force of motion will alter any joint's ROM. Internal factors such as neural facilitation, mechanoreceptor inhibition, or arthrokinetic dysfunctions such as joint misalignment or subluxations can all affect muscular force production and alter joint mechanics and range of motion. Nutritional factors, immune system function, and emotional and psychological issues can also cause variations in joint movement abilities. Environmental factors such as temperature, presence of external loads or forces, and the surface used for a base of support also dramatically influence ROM. Simply stated, any joint for any person can demonstrate variable degrees of available mobility depending on numerous factors.

If even the same joint on the same person can vary under different circumstances, imagine the degree of variance in possible ROM from person to person. The individual genetic differences of anatomical factors such as bone lengths, ligaments, joint capsules, tendons, muscles, and fascia can create a large divergence in estimating what a "normal" ROM should be. There are no "normal" people, only data that suggest what normal may be under conditions identical to the conditions in which the data were gathered. Increased joint mobility, therefore, should be trained at a level based on the needs and goals of each person, with limited comparisons to others. The following are some of the anatomical components that limit joint mobility.

Muscle Limits

Although muscle stiffness or flexibility is often perceived as the major limiting factor, several other anatomical factors contribute to decreased ROM. In fact, muscle and its associated fascia are attributed to less than half of the internal resistance to joint ROM. Healthy muscle (free from adhesions and scarring) is designed with high levels of elasticity, so it should offer only minimal amounts of resistance to joint mobility within normal ranges depending on speed of movement and presence of external forces. Also, since muscle tension is controlled by the sensorimotor system, you must realize that muscle tightness is often a symptom of some other problem. Muscles can intentionally attempt to limit passive and active joint movement as a protective mechanism in order to decrease connective tissue damage and joint wear. This is particularly the case when mechanical issues are associated with the desired joint motion, such as arthrokinetic dysfunctions, muscular inhibition, and muscular imbalances around the joint. Under these conditions, simply stretching the muscles will probably not provide for any prolonged increase in joint mobility and can even cause further degeneration of associated tissue and joint structures.

The most significant way in which the muscles can limit active joint mobility is through active insufficiency. In chapter 1 this was defined as the diminished capacity of a muscle to produce active tension once shortened or lengthened too far. Therefore, active range of motion is limited by the muscle's ability to produce force at certain lengths. This is particularly true for muscles that cross over two or more joints, because they are more prone to active insufficiency when they are either shortened or lengthened over both joints simultaneously. Muscles can also limit active mobility from inhibition, inflammation, prior damage, fatigue, or simply a lack of strength. Active insufficiency is taken into consideration for ROM recommendations in all exercises in this book.

The study of the concurrent force systems that occur with any joint motion reveals another possible limit to joint ROM. The pull of a muscle is always a resultant pull of numerous muscle fibers, all in slightly divergent directions. This means that while a muscle appears to contract in one general direction, it also applies other forces to the joint. The muscle produces a rotational force in one direction in order to move the bone, yet it also generates a translatory force at the joint, most often in another direction. This translatory force compresses the joint, distracts the joint, or increases the shear force across the joint as the joint progresses through a full ROM. Although this may not automatically decrease active joint mobility, comprehension of these facts may influence your choice to purposely limit ROM, particularly for a resistance exercise if the loaded movement can increase risk. Some exercises in this book have been modified in ROM for such reasons.

Skeletal Limits

Once analyzed, it is apparent that the bones are designed in a purposeful manner for a number of individual and combined functions. Each bone's unique construction allows for certain amounts of joint mobility in specific directions while further restricting the movement in other directions. For example, the shallow concave shape of the glenoid fossa (shoulder socket) allows for a great amount of motion for the attached humerus. It is by far the most mobile joint on the human body, allowing an extreme amount of possible movement patterns in numerous directions. However, mobility is restricted when the shoulder is placed in specific positions. For example, once internally rotated, the humerus can be limited in abduction to less than 90 degrees depending on associated scapular movement and scapular type. Movement beyond this range can impinge on certain musculature and the bursa as the humerus begins to compress the tissue against the acromion process of the scapula.

The way in which bones are designed to move collectively also plays a critical role in providing for any movement. Keeping with the example discussed previously, once the shoulder is externally rotated and proper scapular movement is assisting, abduction to 180 degrees may be possible. However, further investigation reveals that for this level of scapular–humeral movement or "rhythm" to occur, there must also be an associated positioning of the spine and rib cage. So here you can see how skeletal design will have a large part in determining overall joint mobility.

Also a look at bony surfaces may reveal other preferences to not only the amount of desirable joint motion but also the position where joint motion is better designed to occur. For example, the hip socket has a much broader surface and a greater degree of articular cartilage on the superior aspect or upper surface than on the posterior aspect or back surface. This analysis clearly shows its design is prepared for supporting weight better in a standing position than in a seated, flexed-hip position. Therefore it is designed to provide for greater amounts of mobility and can better support load when starting from a standing position such as when performing squats than when starting in a seated, flexed-hip position such as when performing a leg press. Here you can see how joint design affects not only mobility but also joint stability. All exercise selections and ROM recommendations in this book are congruent with designed joint structures and joint functions.

Connective Tissue Limits

Another limitation to joint ROM imposed by the musculoskeletal system is from the various other connective tissues. A joint of the body is the meeting place of any two bones. Bones are held together by fibrous tissue known as ligaments. The elasticity of ligaments is low, and they are most definitely not designed to stretch. Any significant stretching incurred to a ligament further than its intended design and short of tearing can cause permanent deformation and reduce its ability to stabilize the joint.

Tendons of a joint complex attach the muscle to the bone and, like ligaments, are also very resistant to stretching. Any lengthening in the muscle–tendon unit typically comes from the muscle itself because tendons are also prone to deformation and tearing if a significant stretching force is applied. In fact, the stretch reflex used to generate additional power for any movement is thought to be a protective mechanism of the muscle–tendon unit to keep it from being stretched too far. This stretch reflex can be used for performance of plyometric movements, so any previous damage to a tendon will likely reduce power and make the joint more prone to injury.

Another component of the joint that affects ROM is the joint capsule. Although the capsule has more elasticity than ligaments or tendons, it also has plastic characteristics that help to stabilize the joint and to transfer forces from a working muscle to the adjacent bone. This means that the joint capsule is also often exposed to a high degree of risk for damage when ROM exceeds its designed limits. Since most of the characteristics of capsules, ligaments, and tendons are predetermined by their structures, research suggests that almost half of the flexibility at any joint is determined by these structures and is related to genetics. In other words, some people are just born with more ROM capabilities than others in their connective tissues. This also means that those who force their joints to limits beyond their genetic potential risk damage and are unlikely to gain functional joint mobility.

Sensorimotor System

Joint mobility is not totally determined by the passive and active systems but is also subservient to the control system. This system includes the mechanisms in which all sensory information is obtained, processed, and transferred back through the spinal cord to the peripheral nervous system. These impulses excite and inhibit the proper concert of muscles in order to produce the desired movement or reaction. The amount of muscle activation the nerves can control varies at different ranges of motion, particularly when confronted with higher levels of resistance. In such cases, it may be better to reduce ROM as well as the resistance rather than train motor patterns that do not efficiently produce the joint ROM desired. ROM can also be enhanced as more neurological control of the muscles is enhanced.

Stretching for Mobility

As most sport and life movements depend more on active ROM than on passive ROM, it is becoming more popular to focus on stretching techniques that promote active stretching over passive stretching. A review of research and contemporary literature suggests that an increase in active ROM not only reduces incidence of injury but also may delay muscle fatigue, decrease muscle soreness, and increase performance. The following are comparative descriptions of both types of stretching

1. Passive stretching, similar to static stretching, involves the use of a force outside the joint for limb or body movement. This force can be gravity, as when simply leaning over to try to touch the toes, as pictured in figure 3.4. A passive stretch can be provided by another person moving the limb or trunk, or it can be done by simply pulling with the arms or with the use of a machine or device. The common element of a passive stretch is that the muscles around the joint are not active in producing the stretching movement. For this reason the benefits of passive stretching are often questioned and are a topic of debate and research. One of the possible advantages to passive stretching is that it can be more relaxing than active stretching. This can help with stress reduction and promote a general awareness of the muscles.

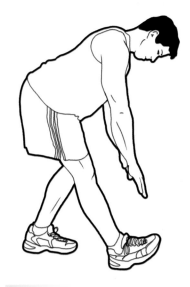

Figure 3.4 Passive stretching.

2. Active stretching, also known as dynamic stretching, is more reliant on the voluntary activation of an agonist muscle group in order to stretch its reciprocal antagonist. An example of this is presented in figure 3.5 as the man simply pulls one leg up off the floor as high as possible against gravity while keeping it locked at the knee and the foot dorsiflexed. This would constitute an active stretch for the hamstrings and gastrocnemius. Similar movements can be done for any muscle group. Active stretching works to strengthen the agonist, helps to reset or reprogram the neuromuscular system, and decreases inhibitory tension of the opposing muscles.

Active stretching tends to be better than passive stretching at increasing the ability to produce active movement, but it is specific to the rate, range, and speed of activation. Therefore there are several methods of performing an active stretch, such as the contract–contract technique shown in figure 3.6. Here, an isometric contraction is performed for the targeted muscle followed by a voluntary contraction of the antagonist muscle group. This active stretching technique is purported to help decrease inhibitory responses within the targeted muscle and also to promote joint stability along with joint mobility.

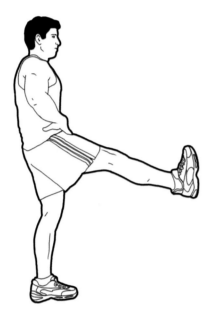

Figure 3.5 Active stretching.

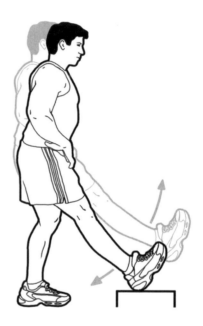

Figure 3.6 Contract–contract technique for active stretching.

3. Passive–active stretching is a combined stretching technique that can involve either contract–relax or relax–contract techniques. Contract–relax requires a partner who assists with a voluntary contraction of the muscle to be stretched followed by a relaxation of the muscle with an immediate assisted passive stretch. This is designed to decrease inhibitory responses of the muscle and is a simplified version of PNF (proprioceptive neuromuscular facilitation). The relax–contract technique involves beginning with a relaxed passive stretch that is held at maximum ROM. This is followed by an active attempt to further ROM. If successful, the new ROM is where the next passive stretch begins, followed again by another active attempt for increased ROM.

4. In progressive–dynamic stretching, the lengthening antagonist muscle is always sensitive to the speed of stretch as well as the amount of stretch. Therefore, developing specific joint ROM at the specific speed and at the specific intensity levels in the specific movement patterns as needed for the life or sport demand would be highly valuable. This combined active and passive type of stretching is characterized by a practice of movement patterns that promotes gradual increases in range, speed, and intensity of motion. This is often not seen as stretching as much as a warm-up but is often performed just before participation in a sporting event and is the most specific type of stretching that can be performed. These rehearsed motor programs facilitate muscle synergy, decrease inhibition, and decrease viscosity of tissue, all of which should help to increase active ROM just before using the movement at full speed.

Performance Abilities

Speed, agility, and power are probably the most sought-after attributes for athletes of all calibers in virtually every sport and are referred to as the performance abilities. However, optimal enhancement of these qualities is dependent on the prior development of the base abilities, as shown in figure 3.1 on page 30. These performance abilities rely on the cohesive and integrated functions of the control, active, and passive systems of the body. The key to developing increased speed, agility, and power comes from high levels of neuromuscular efficiency and a blend of prior increases in specific types of strength, static and dynamic stability, balance, appropriate mobility, and even certain levels of endurance.

Traditionally it was thought that one could improve biomotor abilities separately and then summate them for the desired result. Since the neuromuscular system is highly programmable, it needs the proper input on how each of the specific improved abilities needs to be combined for use in the final program. For example, just because an athlete has improved strength in the gym or speed on the track, increased vertical jump, improved flexibility, mastery of balance exercises, or improved power cleans is no guarantee the athlete will perform better in his given sport, because none of these improvements will transfer specifically. Rather, the athlete must now take these improved abilities and combine them and practice them within the precise motor programs in the proper environments as needed for his sport. Otherwise, these improved abilities lie in wait as nothing more than potential.

Speed

Speed is one of the most difficult biomotor abilities to improve. Its interdependent relationships with mobility, stability, and endurance are often overlooked, and its reliance on strength is more often underestimated. The way in which speed is intended to be expressed or used will determine the specific mix of maximal strength, relative strength, explosive strength, speed strength, and endurance strength that will need to be developed. This relationship between speed and strength is important to remember because some coaches and athletes believe that speed is purely a genetic gift and improving it is next to impossible. This perception is often a result of experiencing failures with running programs that did not devote adequate time to improving strength or used antiquated training techniques.

Genetic factors such as anatomical design, muscle fiber type dominance, biomechanical advantages, and sensorimotor system structure may set certain physiological and neurological limitations for maximal speed potential just as they do for every other biomotor ability. However, this does not mean that significant improvements in current levels of speed are impossible for those who are willing to learn and practice the processes involved in speed improvement.

Research on muscle physiology shows that all muscles are composed of a mixture of different fibers divided into two types: fast twitch and slow twitch. Therefore, people born with a higher proportion of fast-twitch fibers will have a higher potential for maximal speed. However, further research has indicated that there is actually a continuum of several types of muscle fiber ranging from type I (slow-twitch oxidative fiber) to type IIb (fast-twitch glycolytic fiber).

Nine different muscle fiber types and their abilities to adapt to different training stimuli are presented in chapter 6. Research suggests that muscle fibers of the same type can shift their ability to perform slightly different functions in response to training and perhaps be trained to perform better for speed and power demands. This range of adaptability holds promise for increased speed potential but is limited because it is unlikely that type I (slow-twitch oxidative) fibers can ever be trained to perform the same way as type IIB (fast-twitch glycolytic) fibers.

Genetic structures of the control system have also been cited as a barrier to maximal speed. Elite sprinters appear to have more organized central nervous systems. Their bodies often have reticular and spinal cord systems capable of transmitting much higher frequencies of discharges than the average person. In other words, reflexes and commands from all three levels of control are sent at faster and more frequent rates. How much of this is adaptive to their training and participation in competitive events and how much is simply genetics are inconclusive. However, we do know that the control system is programmable and sensitive to training, so improvements in speed related to adaptations of the control system are possible.

Speed and Strength Relationships

Both physiological and neural adaptations that would increase potential for improved maximal speed can be attained through proper training of specific types of strength. Increases in maximal strength, as previously discussed, appear to offer carryover benefits to all types of strength. Increases in maximal strength are due primarily to neurological adaptations and the improved recruitment of fast-twitch fibers. The fast-twitch fibers are the key for speed enhancement because they can produce higher levels of force, produce force at faster rates, and provide for greater power output. Therefore it is logical to assume that gains in maximal strength, particularly within the muscles controlling the trunk and moving the limbs of the body, should give added potential for increased arm and leg movement. Increases in maximal strength developed with the use of general movement patterns such as squatting, lunging, pushing, pulling, and rotating the trunk also have a higher carryover to arm and leg speed development than isolated movement patterns have.

Also, it is important to remember that increases in maximal strength and recruitment of fast-twitch muscle fiber are obtained through greater force demand. With resistance training this means using greater loads, not using faster tempos. Moving weights faster increases rotational inertia and requires exponentially greater levels of effort by the muscles and the control system in order to decelerate the weight and limb. This means that heavier loads cannot be used safely, which limits recruitment of fast-twitch motor units and compromises gains in maximal strength. Moving any object that must be held means that a larger portion of sensorimotor system control is prioritized and directed toward deceleration as opposed to acceleration. This is not conducive to improvement in maximal strength or speed.

Faster tempos of exercise movements free of the need to decelerate an object would, however, be ideal for developing speed strength, which would also be a key type of strength beneficial for achieving greater amounts of arm or leg speed. This type of strength training therefore focuses more on the speed of movement rather than on the amount of resistance. To be fast you must train fast. Though this is not done effectively using weights, other tools are ideal for this type of strength development. Medicine-ball training and target-mitt training can be helpful for developing increased arm and trunk movement speed. Similarly, integrated use of a variety of methods and equipment such as stadium stair sprinting, sprinting in sand, and using weighted sleds and parachutes are all viable methods of improving leg speed for running.

Whether the training priority would lean more on developing starting strength or acceleration strength would depend on the present strengths of the athlete and the demand of the activity. The development of starting strength for starting speed, or quickness, has some importance for any athlete because all speed movements must have a beginning. Athletes who often begin in stationary positions and move within limited distances, such as tennis players, short-distance sprinters, football players, and boxers, are all examples of athletes who would benefit from good levels of starting speed as well as explosive speed, or power. Exercise movements that begin with the muscles in a prelengthened position and techniques that promote a fast initial movement, such as a deadlift or power clean, would be ideal for this type of strength development. Specific positional quickness exercises such as focused work on the first few steps out of a given stance would also be sensible training practices.

Athletes competing in sports that involve constant motion and movement over great distances with accompanying needs for sudden bursts of speed have a greater need for acceleration speed, which is derived from their acceleration strength. *Acceleration* is most simply defined as the process of increasing velocity (speed). Rate of acceleration is often more important than maximal speed for many athletes in order to catch a ball or to overtake an opponent. It is particularly important for athletes competing in field and long-court sports such as football, soccer, rugby, hockey, and basketball. Studies on elite athletes who have comparable maximal speed have demonstrated high degrees of variances in their acceleration speed, suggesting that this component is differentiated and therefore trainable. Resistance training exercises are not as logical for training acceleration speed nor are the use of running sleds or partner-resisted and assisted acceleration training using resistance bands.

For many athletes, increases in relative strength are also important for gaining greater speed. This is a matter of simple physics. The amount of body weight compared to strength will directly affect overall speed more than strength itself. In fact, a reduction of body fat along with a moderate strength increase could do more for achieving greater speed than a high degree of strength gain coupled with no weight loss, depending on the resultant levels of relative strength. A diet and an overall exercise program designed to reduce body fat and maintain muscle are often imperative in these situations.

Endurance strength is an important type of strength when maximal, or close to maximal, speeds are needed to be maintained for longer periods. A long run-back in football and a breakaway run in rugby and soccer are examples of endurance speed derived mostly from established levels of endurance strength. Endurance speed is a continuum representing a ratio of needed speed to endurance; endurance strength is the most prominent where more speed is desired. Long-distance running and swimming events are related more to straight endurance and require less endurance strength. This relationship triangle of strength, speed, and endurance again demonstrates the interdependence of various biomotor abilities and how each person needs his or her unique mix to perform at optimal levels for specific goals.

Speed and Other Biomotor Relationships

Joint mobility is also an important factor for improving speed. The degree and speed of active joint motion in any direction is dependent on both the strength and the pliability of the joint connective tissues and also the extensibility of the antagonist muscles. If connective tissues such as the joint capsule or the antagonist muscles feel a need to limit or halt movement, not only will speed be compromised, but injury is also likely. Remember that these tissues must not only be prepared for the range of movement but also for the speed and force of movement. That is why regular active stretching and progressive dynamic stretching are imperative for performance of high-speed movements. Including this flexibility training as part of a warm-up before practice or participation in high-speed activities is also highly recommended. This prepares not only antagonistic tissue but the entire neuromuscular system as well by recalling and rehearsing motor patterns before activating them at full speed.

Joint stability, particularly dynamic stability, is a necessity for high-speed training or activities. With higher speeds comes eventual higher impact. The word eventual is used because studies of ground forces show significantly less impact on the feet during a full sprint than during a run or jog. This is due to the body's forward momentum and reduced contact with the ground. However, eventually the movement must end and often it is done with a sudden stop that requires great demand for joint stability to help absorb this force and halt the movement. If discussing hand speed as opposed to leg speed, then the same increased need for joint dynamic stability can be observed as speed of motion increases. An example would be a boxer's need for increased dynamic stability from the wrist all the way down to the ankle to absorb the greater impacts associated with faster, more powerful punches. A pitcher's increased need for dynamic stability to assist with deceleration of the arm and trunk after throwing a fastball is another example of the stability-to-speed relationship that is present even for more upper-body-dominated movements.

Speed and Running Mechanics

Speed for any movement relies on optimal intermuscular and intramuscular coordination for the biomechanical control of the trunk and limbs. Mechanical analysis of a running gait as presented in figure 3.7 demonstrates the biomechanical complexity involved in production of running speed. Gait can be broken down into three phases: a stance phase, a swing phase, and a propulsion phase.

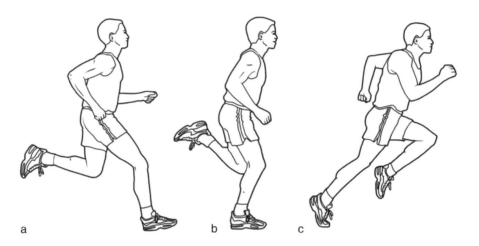

a   b   c

Figure 3.7   Phases of gait; *(a)* stance phase, *(b)* swing phase, and *(c)* propulsion phase.

The stance, or support, phase is signaled by the impact with the ground, which is a heel strike during running or a toe strike when sprinting. The less time spent here, the faster the movement will be and, typically, the fewer associated impact forces due to the increased horizontal momentum. Elastic and kinetic energy are stored in this phase from the eccentric loading of the leg, which will be used in the following phases.

The swing, or recovery, phase is characterized by a pulling action of the leg and a rotation or torque of the pelvis, which begins the use of the stored elastic energy and the transition into the subsequent propulsion phase.

The propulsion, or drive, phase is signaled by the heel lift, the extension of the hip and opposite shoulder, and the actual push off of the ground. Remaining stored energy is released and combined with the forward momentum of the body into a powerful action that propels the body up and forward, creating the stride length between the next impact of the contralateral foot and the beginning of the next stance phase.

Any lack of mobility or breakdown in stability, or reduction of speed strength, explosive strength, or endurance strength during any of these phases of gait not only will affect the speed but also compromise mechanical function, increase metabolic cost, induce muscular compensation, and possibly create faulty motor engrams which are basically stored inefficient motor programs that can lead to injury and increased mechanical wear of the joints.

For the neuromuscular system to consistently produce efficient running or sprinting movements, balanced muscular strength, stability, and mobility all need to be present and maintained. This is why beginning runners may consider running for shorter distances and stopping well before experiencing fatigue in order to establish efficient running technique. Additional conditioning can be done with a variety of other aerobic activities, if needed, until the running distance is gradually increased to the desired amount.

The two measurements of running technique that can be assessed for possible improvements are stride length and stride frequency. Either one can be measured fairly easily and recorded for future comparisons. Realize that an increase in either one at the expense of the other will typically slow maximal speed. Other authors have cited these observations when working with people who were incorrectly taught to overemphasize stride length at the cost of decreased stride frequency.

Research has demonstrated a significant degree of variance between stride length and frequency even when comparing athletes with almost identical maximal speeds. Contemporary opinions among published professionals are leaning toward promoting the use of specific-form running techniques along with regular sprint training to increase speed. These protocols rely more on the adaptability of the neuromuscular system to develop the optimal ratio of stride length to stride frequency for each person's own anatomy as opposed to subjective intervention from the coach.

Power

In the fitness and athletic worlds, power is often expressed as the combination of strength and speed. Power, in fact, is a physics term used as a measurement of work equal to the amount of force multiplied by the rate and typically expressed in watts. Therefore since all movement requires some level of force and is performed at a certain rate, all movements require power. For our purposes and as consistent with the fitness enthusiast's and professional's perception, power will be considered as the ability to generate the appropriate force within the appropriate amount of time. Activities that have a great need for power are quick and explosive movements such as jumping and throwing and swinging movements with implements such as bats, clubs, and rackets. Because the use of stored elastic energy can increase power dramatically, these movements typically integrate the use of a stretch reflex and are reliant on the development of a person's level of explosive strength. However, prerequisite development of other biomotor abilities and specific programming factors of the neuromuscular system are also critical components of optimal power.

To express power, consider Newton's law of inertia, which states that a body at rest or in uniform motion will stay at rest or in uniform motion until acted upon by another force. This means that in order to quickly move your body or an object at rest or while already in motion, its inertia (which is its mass multiplied by its velocity) must be overcome with a quick production of force known as impulse.

Power is derived primarily from a person's level of explosive strength. Explosive strength is developed by learning how to integrate the stretch reflex or use of the stored elastic energy coupled with fast, voluntary concentric actions of the muscles to quickly propel the body or accelerate the limbs. Explosive strength is needed for quick changes of direction and for powerful movements such as jumping and throwing. Sports such as volleyball, basketball, football, and baseball all have frequent demands for explosive strength. Several resistance training exercises, such as Olympic lifts, cleans, and snatches, are often prescribed for the development of explosive strength and power.

Technically, however, these exercise movements may be better suited for development of starting strength because the primary muscles always begin in a prelengthened position. Exercises with tempos (such as a squat at a 1011 tempo; see chapter 4, page 63, for an explanation of the meaning of this four-digit number) that promote a quick eccentric movement followed by a quick concentric movement with no pause between should do well for development of explosive strength. Plyometric exercises would be even more appropriate because the athlete would train with the specific amount of load (that is, the athlete's own body weight) and can train more directionally and positionally specific to the event demand. Remember, no sport other than weightlifting requires moving fast with weights.

Power improvements would be beneficial not only for athletes but also for improved safety and quality of life for anyone. Power is needed for activities such as bounding up a flight of stairs, swinging your body over a fence, and jumping to safely avoid an oncoming car. Even less extreme possible life demands such as throwing a bag of trash into a high receptacle, quickly altering gait movement to regain balance, and rising quickly from a chair also require some level of power. Power should be trained and progressed gradually according to the current abilities of the person and with the end result in mind. In other words, there will be an increased risk with limited benefit for attempting to train the average person to develop the levels of power needed by the elite athlete.

Plyometric Training for Power

The term *plyometric training* comes from the naturally occurring plyometric actions of a muscle during movements such as running and jumping. The natural stretch–shortening cycle of muscle contraction has a naturally occurring reflex termed the *myotatic stretch reflex,* which can produce more power when used along with an appropriate voluntary contraction of the muscle. The mechanisms of the stretch reflex are highly detailed and involve the integrated functions of the control, active, and passive systems. The stretch reflex is believed to be a designed function of the neuromuscular system for self-protection and for mechanical efficiency. The following is a summary of the science behind plyometric training.

As a muscle is eccentrically loaded during what is termed the *amortization phase,* particularly when done with high velocity or speed, elastic energy is immediately stored in the tendon and serial elastic components of the muscle for the subsequent concentric action. The mechanical delay period between eccentric and concentric muscle contraction is the coupling time and is a far shorter period than the time it would take to activate any voluntary contraction through cognitive control. Immediately following the eccentric stretch is the forceful concentric contraction known as the summation phase. Combining this stretch–reflex muscle contraction with the appropriate voluntary movement produces a much more powerful movement than could have been created through a voluntary contraction on its own.

Various jump training, speed training, and medicine-ball exercises can be used for enhancing the use of the stretch reflex and developing the potential for increased power. Figure 3.8a depicts a plyometric exercise that can be used for targeting development of the anterior oblique subsystem. It emphasizes the action of the swing phase of gait. Likewise, figure 3.8b could be used for targeting the posterior oblique subsystem and emphasizes action of the propulsion phase of gait. Figures 3.9a, 3.9b, and 3.9c are medicine-ball tosses used for developing explosive strength of the core muscles that use and therefore train the general movement patterns of flexion, extension, and rotation, respectively.

Numerous books, such as Donald Chu's *Jumping Into Plyometrics,* provide a variety of exercises that can be strategically selected based on the desired goals of the person, such as sport-specific training. Chapter 5 of this book also provides more information on targeting subsystems and training general movement patterns. By analyzing the general movement patterns most used by a particular athlete, and determining the subsystems most needed for training, you can customize a resistance training program to include specific plyometric and agility exercises to enhance the athlete's athletic potential.

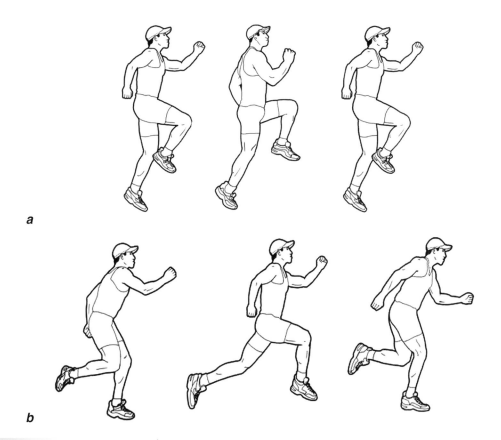

Figure 3.8 *(a)* The swing phase and *(b)* the propulsion phases of training.

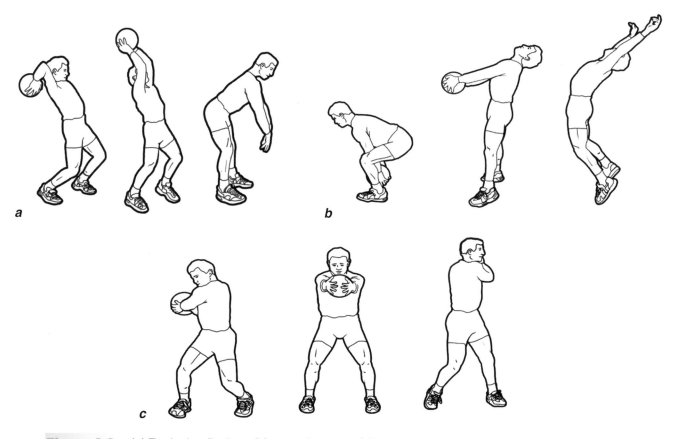

Figure 3.9 *(a)* Explosive flexion, *(b)* extension, and *(c)* rotation.

Progression Toward Plyometrics

Plyometric training requires the body to deal with high levels of impact force or high amounts of torque force applied to the spine. The stabilization and eccentric deceleration demands are much higher than most people realize or have properly prepared for. Some experts have suggested that a person should exhibit the abilities to squat 10 repetitions in 10 seconds with 1.5 times the person's body weight before aggressively engaging in plyometric training. The person must also exhibit optimal spinal flexion, extension, and particularly rotation abilities as well as strength while under load in a controlled setting before engaging in aggressive medicine-ball training. These recommendations may sound too restrictive but actually only provide a hint of the exponentially increased amount of forces that will be handled by the joints and spine to efficiently and safely adapt to traditional plyometric and medicine ball training.

A possible basic progression toward jump training could begin with simply training the body to statically stabilize a squat position. Possible static loading followed by loaded squat movements at slow and controlled tempos with pauses would promote more static strength gains and develop starting strength and maximal strength. You could implement progression to squat movements with lighter loads and faster tempos in order to develop explosive strength. After that, the gradual introduction of plyometric exercises could begin, assuming no limitations have emerged. Even Chu stated in his book, *Jumping Into Plyometrics,* that plyometric training should be considered as the "icing" on a cake. I believe that cake should be comprised of the proper mix of the ingredients—strength, endurance, stability, and mobility—that are derived from a sound base biomotor development program.

Agility

Agility is difficult to define because it is the culmination of nearly all other biomotor abilities. I choose to define it as the outward display of the person's level of neuromuscular efficiency, which means the ability of the neuromuscular system to efficiently store, recall, combine, execute, monitor, and modify multiple motor programs as needed to produce the desired movements.

Agility is often the most important biomotor ability for athletes to improve for enhanced performance within their sports. The constant stopping, starting, and changing of direction involved in most sports incorporate power with speed and demand quick changes of force output and integration of different types of strength, high amounts of stability, good balance, and proper amounts of mobility. Endurance is also needed if agility is required for prolonged periods, which applies to most athletes at some level. Maximal levels of speed, power, strength, endurance, or joint mobility are rarely as important for success in most sports as having the optimal mix and coordination of all these, which is what makes up a person's agility.

Agility and Coordination

Neuromuscular coordination is a continual process necessary for the demonstration of agile movement. All the related systems for improved intermuscular and intramuscular control, increased reflex activity, and faster responses to feedback from afferent receptor information require practice and repeated exposure to the stimuli. Neuromuscular coordination for increased agility is refined through the three basic stages as identified in chapter 1 in the section titled Neuromuscular Efficiency and Motor Learning (page 17).

As any movement pattern is practiced and refined, modifications are developed and also stored for more efficient recall when needed again. In time, movement patterns that once required high levels of voluntary thought and cognitive control become more reliant on proprioception and move toward automated control. As with all biomotor abilities, the genetic structure and sensorimotor capabilities are different for each person. Consequently, some people will need more practice than others for neuromuscular efficiency and agility to develop and may never reach the abilities of others no matter how well and often they practice.

Agility Training

Training for agility should be preceded by development of all base abilities and perhaps even some forms of power training. Specific types of strength development, adequate endurance, as well as the optimal proportion of joint stability and mobility are needed for safe and efficient agility training. Any muscular weakness, low endurance, joint stiffness or joint laxity, and lack of power will not only hamper agility but also increase the likelihood of injury when attempting to perform movements requiring high levels of neuromuscular coordination.

Both agility and power exercises should be trained according to the SAID principle, which stands for *s*pecific *a*daptations to the *i*mposed *d*emands. This means that improved power and agility developed in any exercise movement will transfer only in proportion to the similarities between the environment and conditions in which they were developed and those in which you wish to later perform them. And even then, only through sport-specific practice will they truly be integrated and have any potential for increasing athletic performance.

Muscle Hypertrophy

For many people the driving motivation for engaging in resistance training has little to do with improved health or biomotor ability and performance enhancement. Rather, it is fueled by the desire to achieve aesthetic goals. Probably the most common aesthetic goal people strive to achieve through resistance training is muscular hypertrophy, though they may not phrase it as such. Gains in muscle size (often stated as mass, increased tone, contour, shaping, or even increased muscle definition) are actually various levels of muscle hypertrophy combined with some level of fat reduction. Therefore, as a professional trainer or strength coach, you should first understand some basic truths on what muscle hypertrophy is before you attempt to achieve it for yourself or supply it for others.

First realize that hypertrophy of muscle is a reactive and protective adaptation of the body; it is a response to repetitive joint and muscle stress. Therefore you can see that to gain more hypertrophy, you must first apply and then be able to adapt to greater levels and volumes of stress. From this realization you can also see that hypertrophy is limited and proportionally temporary. However, other effects of the increased stress may be of a more permanent nature, such as connective tissue damage or joint deterioration. Hypertrophy is a side effect of neuromuscular stress that does not necessarily improve performance or health of the body. And once stress levels are reduced or sometimes even just efficiently adapted to, then muscle size most likely will decrease.

Hypertrophy and Strength

Hypertrophy is not a neurological adaptation but rather a structural change in tissue size and density as a result of primarily metabolic adaptations in response to frequent imposed demands. As such, it is often believed that there is no direct relationship between increases in muscle size and muscle strength. However, further investigation reveals that an increase in cross-sectional muscle mass will provide for mechanical advantages that result in greater muscular force output. Also, the increase in muscle size is attributed in part to the increase in the size and number of contractile proteins within the myofibrils. The increase in heavy-chain myosin size and increased number of associated actin filaments provide for more potential cross-bridging, which will in turn provide for greater levels of force production. Therefore, you can conclude that there is good reason to expect some level of strength increase along with hypertrophy, which may be an important goal for some people.

Hypertrophy and Fat Loss

Changes in overall levels of muscle mass also have a significant effect on a person's metabolism and caloric expenditures. In fact, the loss of muscle mass is a primary contributing factor to decreased metabolic demand and increased body fat in the process of aging. Therefore, hypertrophy has a direct long-term effect on maintenance or decreases in body fat, while resistance training (which is the activity best suited for gaining hypertrophy) also provides for immediate contributions to fat loss. Resistance training can burn a significant amount of calories in a single session, which will assist in fat loss, particularly when done in a circuit-type sequence that allows for little rest and high cardiorespiratory demands. Also, the related hormonal responses, such as increased testosterone and growth hormone release that often accompanies resistance training, can elevate metabolic activity for several hours after the session. These findings explain why people who have greater amounts of muscle mass and regularly engage in resistance training typically have fewer struggles with maintaining or reducing present levels of body fat than those people who carry less muscle and choose to engage solely in aerobic activity.

Whether the primary adaptations desired from resistance training and an overall exercise program is based on enhancement of one's performance or improvement of one's aesthetics, it is important that you not think of these as exclusive goals. In other words, any program that would develop one with a high cost to the other would not typically be considered successful in the eyes of most clients or athletes. Certain performance goals may actually involve a change in one's body that may not be viewed as an aesthetic improvement, such as significant gains in muscle or fat. However, the trainer or strength coach should make every attempt to keep this trade-off within reasonable levels to insure the overall health and well-being of their client or athlete. Conversely, the pursuit of aesthetic goals should never result in significant or permanent deficiencies in performance or result in injury. Information on designing exercise programs to balance both development of biomotor abilities for enhancement of performance and achieving aesthetic goals will be provided in the next part of this book.

Technique and Programming

Part II presents theories on resistance training exercise technique, exercise selection, and exercise programming based on human structure, function, and adaptation. Here you can apply the information presented in part I and understand how to choose and implement safe and effective techniques and modify any exercise to meet the needs and abilities of each person you train.

In part II you will also learn how to arrange all selected exercises into efficient and challenging daily training routines that are part of well-designed and tailored training programs. This part also presents a thought process on creating systems for manipulating all programming variables—intensity, volume, frequency, duration, and sequence—in order to achieve the goals and address the needs of each client and athlete you train.

The actual program examples provided are for teaching purposes only and are not intended to be directly applied or used by any particular person. They do, however, embody and demonstrate every principle related to exercise selection and programming presented in part II. These examples will help you understand how to use exercise selection and sequencing to design purposeful training routines to form the foundation of the overall program.

Through careful study, you can also see how program variables are systematically manipulated during each phase of the mesocycle in order to promote the desired adaptations and develop specific biomotor abilities. Changes in intensity, sets, reps, and tempo are consistent with the physiological factors involved in developing greater levels of muscular endurance, strength, hypertrophy, speed, and power. Again, the examples in this text are for teaching purposes only; they do not reflect any specific person's goals and certainly cannot take into account each person's needs.

Resistance Training Technique

To make any exercise as efficient and as safe as possible, the specific exercise technique used is the most critical variable. I choose the word *variable* because there are numerous opinions and philosophies related to resistance training technique. Several elements constitute technique, and the way in which they are perceived will dictate the overall performance of an exercise. Many resistance exercise techniques presented today were developed in the gym through trial and error. They were approached with predetermined goals, such as the desire to gain more muscle mass or move heavier weight loads. It is apparent that the study of functional anatomy, actual biomechanics, and even simple physics was given little regard in the developmental years of resistance training.

The human body is composed of highly integrated systems. The body is not constructed simply for aesthetic appeal, nor is it designed to just lift heavy weights. Instead it is designed to produce a high variability of movement, specifically movement within the environment of this planet. The active (muscular) system communicates information and responds to reflex actions and commands through its relationship with the control (sensorimotor) system. In turn it works to control the passive (skeletal) system in order to provide stability and movement of the body and outside objects. Therefore exercise technique is extremely critical because we not only stress the hardware of the body with resistance training, we also program the software.

Technique is also the key for receiving the greatest amount of benefit while also reducing the risk associated with any resistance exercise selected. Following are the seven interdependent elements of exercise technique that can be applied to any resistance exercise selected. Each of these elements is explored in this chapter.

1. Goal identification
2. Exercise motion
3. Alignment
4. Positioning
5. Stabilization
6. Tempo
7. Breathing

Goal Identification

Clearly identifying the goal is probably the most important element of technique and should also be done before selecting the exercise itself. The same goals that inspired the exercise selection will also affect all other elements of technique. Modifications in the movement, tempo, alignment, positioning, and stabilization strategies will often need to be made in order to accomplish the desired goals. However, when making any modifications of technique to an exercise, you must still consider biomechanical factors and keep the modifications within the anatomical limits and abilities of the person performing them.

The first part of goal identification may be to decide whether the exercise will enhance performance of the body in some way or is more for achieving an aesthetic change. This does not mean that an exercise would not provide benefits at some level for both types of goals, but rather that you should identify a priority. You would use an entirely different thought process for selecting exercises and allocating technique options to accomplish performance-based goals versus aesthetic-based goals. The focus, desired movement pattern, positioning, and stabilization strategies all should be consistent with the desired goal. Table 4.1 compares the different thought processes involved with performance- and aesthetic-based goals relative to technique options for a selected exercise.

By studying this table you can see how goal identification will determine several elements of technique. For pursuit of a performance-based goal, the focus is on increasing neuromuscular control rather than developing muscular hypertrophy. When selecting compound (multiple-joint) movement exercises for a performance-based goal, you would logically tend to select exercises in accordance with the movement pattern it produces rather than the muscles it may target. Isolated joint exercises selected for a performance-based goal often are done to address a specific muscle weakness or correct a muscular imbalance as opposed to simply isolating a muscle in order to increase its size.

Many performance exercises are performed in asymmetrical positions such as on one leg or in lunge positions and typically offer little, if any, outside stabilization. This increases proprioceptive activity and requires more neural demand for processing of mechanoreceptor feedback and the formulation of motor commands to control the numerous joints and recruit the proper concert of muscle action needed for performance of the movement. Conversely, many aesthetic-based exercises typically offer high amounts of external support and use bilateral movement patterns, making stability less of a challenge and providing less proprioceptive activity. However, where this may be considered a deficit may also be considered a benefit because of the greater amount of neural availability. With less demand on the neural system for providing stability, there is a greater ability to provide for maximal motor unit recruitment of the targeted muscles. This may be ideal for isolating specific muscles for loading and achieving higher amounts of volume in order to gain muscle hypertrophy.

TABLE 4.1 Training Goals and Exercise Technique

Goal	Focus	General movements	Isolated movements	Positioning	Stabilization	Proprioception/ neural demand
Performance based	Enhancing neuromuscular control	Targets movement patterns	Specific strengthening; unilateral	Asymmetryical	Internally stabilized	High proprioception, low neural availability
Aesthetic based	Enhancing muscular size	Targets muscles	Specific hypertrophy; bilateral	Symmetrical	Externally stabilized	Low proprioception, high neural availability

It is not the purpose of this comparison to say that one type of goal is superior to another. In fact, because most people have both performance and aesthetic goals, a good exercise program will provide the appropriate proportion of exercises that address all of a client's goals in accordance with present needs and abilities. Achieving the proper balance of these two often-opposing goals is a difficult task to manage for certain people. For others whose priorities rest predominantly on one side or the other, exercise selection and program design may be more clearly defined yet still is never easy. Chapter 6 provides more information and sample routines that demonstrate possible methods for selecting exercises, modifying techniques, and manipulating program variables to provide for a relative balance for both types of goals. These are supplied only for learning purposes and are not designed specifically for anyone.

Exercise Motion

Probably the element of technique that varies the most in resistance training technique is the exercise motion itself. The exercise motion dictates the use of all individual joints, the recruitment of all involved muscles, and the specific motor patterns to be learned. Therefore the type, path, range, and specificity of motion are all critical factors of exercise technique.

Type and Path of Motion

Four types of movement, or four pathways through which an object may travel, can be attributed to any object. Therefore human movement can be specified according to these classifications.

- *Rotary* motion is the movement of an object or segment around a fixed axis in a curved path. For the purposes of this book, any isolated joint movement where the joint itself is not in motion would be considered a rotatory movement. However, no joint is perfectly rounded, so it technically would be classified as curvilinear movement.

- *Translatory,* or *linear,* motion is the movement of an object or segment in a fixed or linear path. Since all individual joints rotate, they cannot produce linear motion without the cocommitment of another joint. The human body does not produce true linear movement very efficiently. Therefore, consider using free weights or cable equipment for performance of linear path exercises because they will allow for the minor shifts in joint motions and reduce some unnecessary shearing and compressive forces.

- *Curvilinear* motion is the combination of rotary and linear motion. Technically, since no joint of the body is constructed as completely rounded or flat, all human joint motion is curvilinear. As the joint rotates over or glides along bony articular surfaces, slight shifts in the axis results in a curvilinear movement of the distal end of the segment. However, as mentioned previously, for the purposes of this book all individual joint motions will be considered rotary motion.

- *Transrotational* motion, or *general plane* motion, is the rotary movement of a segment around an axis that is also in movement in the same plane. An example of this is the wheel on a moving bicycle. Many of the traditional exercise movements, whether rotary or linear, tend to begin and end in the same general plane of motion. This is often necessary for maintaining the load on the targeted muscle.

It is possible, and may be beneficial for specific goals, to purposely move a joint through two or more planes of movement with a resistance exercise, provided the alignment of the resistance allows for these changes. However, when performing any multiple-plane movement exercise, you need to consider the weakest point of each part of the movement when selecting load. Careful analysis of joint actions and force alignments is also advisable.

Range of Motion

One of the most debated issues in resistance training is range of motion. It has been traditionally believed that training with a full range of motion (ROM) is what brings about the most benefits for muscle and joint performance. The problem here is determining what *full* actually means. For many people, ROM for a specified exercise is perceived as how far the bar or weight load moved. This view often leads to drastic differences in range of actual joint motion from one person to the next because of differences in limb length. Therefore, ROM recommendations should relate to the bar, machine, or other implement.

Several anatomical factors of the joints themselves directly limit safe range of controlled motion, such as the specific shape of the bone endings that involve the joint, bony protuberances, joint articular cartilage, fibrocartilage, and connective tissue (joint capsules and ligaments). Muscle force capabilities such as force angle and length–tension ratios will also influence joint motion, particularly when resisted. This is particularly true for two joint muscles that have become actively insufficient because of extreme shortening or lengthening and can also be inhibited from tension in antagonist muscles. These anatomical limits along with other issues affecting joint ROM are described in chapter 3 in the section titled Mobility. Review of this section along with the information on joint structure in chapter 1 will help you to better understand many of the factors to consider when recommending a specific ROM for any resistance exercise and clearly show why more is not necessarily better.

Specificity of Motion

Equally important as the type and range of motion is the specificity of the motion when it comes to exercise selection and technique. Simply put, the motion should best accomplish the goal, whether performance based or aesthetic based. If the match of movement pattern relative to goal is efficient, then specificity of motion has been accomplished. All exercises are simply a combination of joint movements. For certain performance-based goals, improving the movement pattern itself may be more important than targeting the muscles that produce the movement. Though rarely does any resistance exercise directly transfer to any life or sport movement exactly, it is possible to select exercises with general movement patterns that transfer better to normal life or sport-specific demands. Inclusion of general movement patterns in an exercise program would make sense for most people. Additional specific movement patterns that may better transfer to certain performance needs or best accomplish a specific aesthetic-based goal would also make sense to include in a resistance training program. Remember the SAID principle: specific adaptation to the imposed demand. This means that the body will always attempt to adapt to every aspect of a physiological, neurological, and even psychological stress encountered. Therefore you must also consider the alignment, positioning, stabilization, and even the environment in which you brace yourself or work as well as the movements themselves to fully assess the specificity of the exercise motion.

Alignment

All forces in the universe can be broken down to their core physics and classified into either a pushing force or a pulling force. Alignment is the correct matching of these two forces. Muscle physiology demonstrates that a muscle–tendon unit can only contract or shorten. This action is classified as a pulling force. Therefore, all muscles can only pull, and none can push. The only way to lengthen a muscle is through the active shortening of the antagonistic muscles or from the application of an outside force. For the purposes of this text, alignment is defined as matching the pull of the muscles in opposition to the pull or push of the resistance.

The muscles pull on the bones, which in turn act as a series of levers that can either pull objects toward you or, through the proper combination of pulls, create a pushing force that moves objects away from you. For achieving optimal alignment, understand the fact that all pushes the body creates are in actuality the combined pull of two or more joint actions. For example, the positioning of the hands on a barbell chest press affects the alignment of pulling forces. This pressing movement is a pull of the pectorals and deltoids to horizontally adduct the humerus combined with the pull of the triceps to extend the elbow. Therefore, you must determine which set of pulls are desired to be challenged the most and position the hands accordingly.

As with any other elements of technique, alignment is always interdependent with the goals. Keep in mind that since alignment deals with force application, you should not compromise the integrity of the musculoskeletal system for the pursuit of any goal. For instance, if choosing different feet positions for targeting different contributions of hip and leg muscles on a squat or pressing movement, understand the joints' limits and risks for these different positioning options as well.

Typically, to maintain a balance of efficiency and safety, alignment options are limited to small adjustments in order to slightly skew force application. This can be done for a desired effect or to simply get a variation of inter- and intramuscular recruitment patterns. Slight intentional alignment options can be applied that may not seem the most efficient for increasing one element of technique, such as ROM, but the adjustments challenge and improve another element, such as stabilization.

Alignment is dependent not only on the identified goal but on all other elements of technique as well. For example, to align the opposing forces, you must first know the type and path of motion you desire to perform and compare this to the direction of resisted motion provided by the resistance. Then, to accomplish the desired alignment, proper positioning must take place along with the stabilization necessary for maintaining alignment. Even breathing techniques and the tempo of an exercise can shift alignment during an exercise, making it less efficient.

Positioning

Positioning is another general term often used to convey various meanings. In this text, positioning is the precise manner in which you choose to set the body and place all of its segments before and during any resisted exercise. Positioning is interdependent on the goals involved for selecting the exercise motion itself, and it goes hand in hand with alignment. Maintenance of proper positioning relies on stability and balance and can also be affected by breathing and tempo.

Positioning of the Spine

During any resistance training exercise, it is important to consider the positioning of every joint of the body from the ground up. The most critical segments are the pelvis and spine. The spine is the primary component of the axial skeleton and, along with the attached rib cage and pelvis, provides the main support structure of the body. The spine also houses the spinal cord, which is part of the central nervous system and is the key communication line from the brain to the rest of the body, including vital organs and glands.

The unique structure of the spinal column provides not only support but also mobility through all three planes of movement. These combined roles make the spine an important consideration in resistance training exercises as well as a critical component for the execution of most life or sport movements where both roles are required simultaneously.

Optimal Posture

Other than exercises for targeting the outer trunk musculature and movements designed specifically for improving spinal motion, all other resistance training exercises will position the spine in what is called *optimal posture*. When the spine is positioned in optimal posture it appears to be straight, but in actuality, barring any structural deviations, it maintains certain degrees of its natural curvatures. Optimal posture for resistance training stabilizes the spine with the natural concave lordotic curvatures in the lumbar and cervical regions in place. Only a slight straightening effect and reduction of the convex kyphotic curvature of the thoracic region are noticeable in optimal posture when compared to neutral posture. This is in response to the slightly increased retraction of the scapula and associated extension of the thoracic region in order to better stabilize the spine from flexing under load.

Optimal posture provides for optimal structural and functional efficiency of the entire kinetic chain. It promotes optimal length–tension and force-coupling relationships of all the muscles originating from the torso, pelvis, hip, and shoulder girdle. This directly affects the strength and function of all these associated muscles, which in turn affect the function and synergistic actions of all other muscles and joint movements of the body. The farther the spine travels in any direction from optimal posture, the less mobility it has available in all other directions of movement and the less stable it may become. Figure 4.1 depicts the spine in optimal posture compared to varied positions.

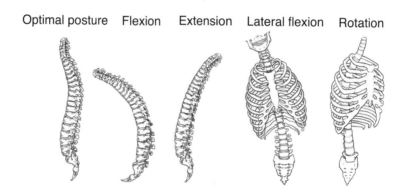

Optimal posture   Flexion   Extension   Lateral flexion   Rotation

Figure 4.1   Optimal posture and spinal positioning.

As the spine moves, length–tension relationships between agonists and antagonists change, which further reduce their ability to stabilize or produce force. All loaded spinal movement also decreases vertebral space and increases disc compression. This does not mean that all movement or disc compression is bad; in fact, vertebral discs rely on compression forces from spinal movement for obtaining nutrients. However, it is important to remember that spinal movement, particularly passive movement under load or at high speeds, often results in exponentially increased degrees of compressive forces on the affected discs, which can dramatically increase the level of risk of the exercise and should be evaluated compared to the relative benefits of the exercise in relation to all training goals.

Spinal positioning must also be accompanied by pelvic positioning. Other than sacroiliac (SI) joint movement, there is no pelvic movement possible without accompanying movement of the spine. An anterior tilt of the pelvis is actually lumbar extension coupled with hip flexion, while a posterior pelvic tilt is simply the result of lumbar flexion coupled with hip extension. Optimal spinal and pelvic positioning is not only important during resistance exercise but also often during normal life movements. Figures 4.2 and 4.3 compare similar high-risk and reduced-risk spinal positioning options relative to loaded flexion for both resistance exercise and everyday movements.

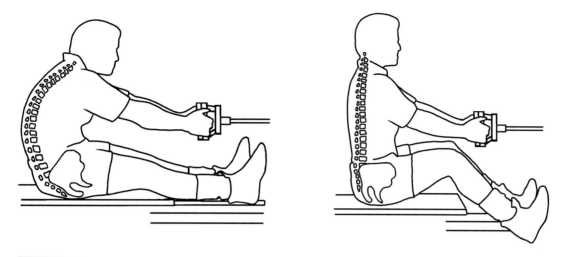

Figure 4.2 High-risk and reduced-risk positioning for resistance training.

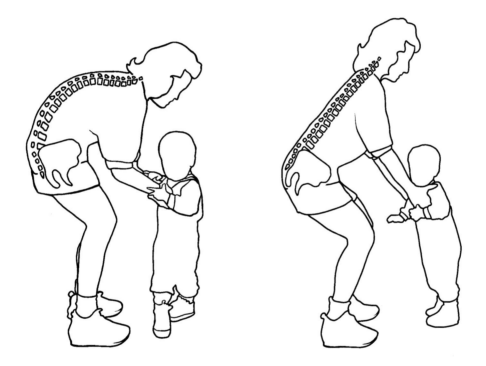

Figure 4.3 High-risk and reduced-risk positioning for everyday movements.

Positioning Options for Various Goals

At times changes of positioning can be made as long as they do not significantly disturb the alignment of forces, are still efficient for performing the desired motion, do not compromise any part of the musculoskeletal system, and can be efficiently stabilized. These optional positioning choices are often used for accomplishing various specific goals in a training phase. For example, a one-arm dumbbell row can be performed in a variety of positions for accomplishing different training goals (figure 4.4).

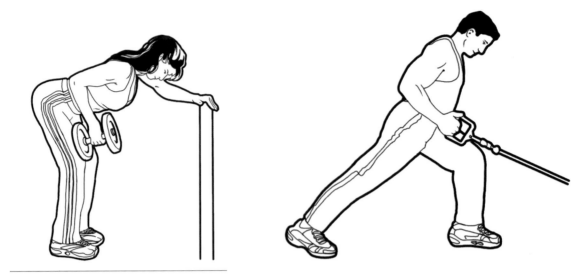

Figure 4.4 Positioning options for accomplishing different goals.

The first positioning option places the body in a symmetrical stance with the arm braced, which provides for more support for stabilization. This positioning may be appropriate for a beginner who needs the additional support or perhaps ideal for the advanced lifter working with maximal loads during a heavy strength phase of the training cycle.

The second positioning option places the body in a lunge position with no external support. This position will require a much higher demand of the gluteal and quadriceps muscles of the forward leg for support and has a higher demand for stabilization and balance. This positioning option also will add torque on the spine and pelvis, which would require increased demand on the posterior oblique subsystem and other associated trunk, pelvic, and hip muscles.

Either option may be selected for different people or for the same person during different phases of training to best accomplish specific training goals. The risk-to-benefit ratio could also be considered equal depending on the selected loads and the abilities of the person and assuming optimal posture, pelvic positioning, and proper alignment are maintained during the exercise movement. Similar comparisons on positioning options can be drawn for any exercise movement or for any muscle group.

Stabilization

Stabilization is the internal ability to control all desired movement or nonmovement of the body and its segments in response to the environment and changes in center of gravity. Stabilization of any joint may be classified as a static demand or a dynamic demand; all exercises require combinations of both and also have some level of balance demand. See chapter 3, in the sections titled Static Stability and Dynamic Stability (page 35), for explanations on the two types of stability.

Balance Demands

Balance is definitely an intricate part of stability. Balance is the process of maintaining center of gravity within the body's base of support. Balance relies predominantly on the activation of specialized reflex actions that vary from the small shifting responses of the ankle or hip in order to balance in place to stepping strategies and associated upper-extremity movement to regain center of gravity and avoid falling while on the move. As presented in chapter 3, balance reflex

diaphragm through an overemphasis of constant transverse abdominal activation will often induce compensational actions of the scalenes, levator scapulae, and other muscles of the cervical spine in an attempt to further elevate the rib cage for achieving greater lung volume. This in turn alters cervical spine positioning and increases mechanical wear. Nerve and vascular structures can also become restricted, leading to muscular dysfunction and reduced blood flow to the upper extremities, as mentioned previously.

Breathing Relationships

Breathing has an obvious relation to stability but can affect other elements of technique as well. Because breathing affects posture, positioning is closely linked to the ability to perform proper and consistent breathing mechanics. If stability and positioning are compromised as a result of faulty breathing methods, then alignment may also be compromised, the motion will then be altered, and accomplishing the training goal will not be possible at the optimal level. Breathing coincides with tempo, so it must be adjusted depending on the tempo demands of the exercise and the phase of the training cycle. In short, practice of efficient breathing methods is a critical element of exercise technique. Inefficient breathing patterns can also increase heart rate and reduce oxygen supply to the muscles and brain, increasing risks and reducing overall performance.

Trainer Techniques

As important as knowing how to perform safe and efficient lifting technique is knowing how to train others to do so. In health clubs and weight rooms you will often see a client or athlete either straining hard to complete a repetition or effortlessly pounding out multiple reps while the trainer or coach leans against the machine, simply counting reps or staring across the room. In either case, they seem totally oblivious to the person's form or technique and offer no advice or actions to correct it. This is not a rare scene; it is often the norm.

Many times trainers and coaches are highly experienced and well versed in exercise sciences, but they were never taught how to instruct others. This next section is a summary that represents only a fraction of the information trainers should know and practice to be the most effective trainers or coaches possible. However, in my experience this may be the most important information for trainers and coaches to learn. Practicing these techniques with passion and consistency will help set you apart and bring about more success than all the knowledge on exercise selection, exercise technique, and exercise programming can ever do. The following five training techniques can be viewed as basic job requirements of anyone responsible for another person's safety during resistance training.

1. Instruct. Provide continued instruction not only on what to do on but how to do it and why. Instruction should be educational yet understandable and meaningful to the client or athlete. Include personal demonstration when possible, because visual learning is probably the most powerful instructional tool available.

2. Coach. Provide immediate and continued feedback on performance throughout each set. Coaching is more about the verbal tips provided relative to correcting form than it is about being a critic or a cheerleader. Coaching should be energetic but not loud and aggressive; positive, not demeaning; and motivational but not insincere.

3. Monitor. Provide a hands-on technique in order to feel, help, and position or stabilize the person's body and guide actual joint motion. Small shifts and compensations can often be felt by the trained hand before becoming visible to the eye. Some courses offer hands-on training to teach monitoring skills.

4. Cue. This is also a hands-on skill that provides proprioceptive cues for the client or athlete while also assisting you, the trainer, with gathering feedback on neuromuscular activity. With experience, you can actually feel the level of tension in a working muscle in order to determine its relative involvement in the exercise. In time, you will also be able to detect muscular fatigue as it begins to set in and can learn to feel for tight protective muscles and weak inhibited muscles, which can all be vital information.

5. Spot. This is the role of assisting or resisting the exercise movement through hands-on manipulation of the load or through providing support directly to the person's body or limbs. Optional spotting positions and methods can be done for any exercise and may be performed differently for each person trained.

Many of the recommended spotting tips along with suggested monitoring and cueing tips that are provided for each exercise in this book require actual touching of the client. It is not the intention to imply that these Trainer Techniques are absolutes or that there are not other optional methods for spotting, monitoring, and cueing that do not require touching that may prove to be effective. Each client and each trainer will have different levels of comfort and different responses to touching. It has been my experience that a professional trainer can learn to gradually implement the hands-on techniques presented herein at the appropriate rate and comfort level of the individual that will help improve the safety and efficiency of every exercise movement performed. However, all trainers will need to take responsibility in deciding how much and in what manner they use these or similar spotting, monitoring, and cueing techniques for each client or athlete they train.

Resistance Exercise Selection

Exercise technique has been presented as the most important variable in exercise programming. A close second is the need for effective exercise selection. In fact, a case could be made that since exercise selection must precede the application of any exercise technique, it may be of equal or even greater importance. It is also evident that even an exercise performed with the most efficient and safest technique possible will still offer only limited value if the exercise was a poor selection in the first place. Therefore exercise selection and technique must go hand in hand.

Appropriate exercise selection is also the key component for building exercise routines and therefore designing effective exercise programs. This entire chapter is dedicated to providing information and developing a thought process for exercise selection. The exercise selection process involves the following four steps that are described further in this chapter.

1. Determining goals
2. Targeting desired movements
3. Targeting desired muscle groups
4. Determining risks versus benefits of selection

Determining Goals

Although a person may have numerous possible combinations of needs and goals that drive their decisions to engage in resistance training, for the purpose of resistance exercise selection we will group goals into two general classifications, performance-based goals and aesthetic-based goals. As you gather stated goals from the client and discover the client's needs from an assessment, you can begin to identify and prioritize training goals and needs. This process not only is vital for effective exercise selection but also will aid in organizing exercises into training routines and designing overall programs as presented in chapter 6. These goals also influence the choices and application of all elements of technique as discussed in chapter 4.

Performance-Based Goals

In short, performance based goals relate to desires for increased joint, muscle, and body control or enhancement of biomotor abilities. Biomotor abilities such as strength, endurance, stability, mobility, speed, power, and agility are the general adaptations or benefits the body can derive from resistance training and other forms of purposeful exercise. Goals associated with performance and increases in biomotor ability can range from simply wanting to tie one's own shoes without back pain to trying to set a world record in a specific event.

Many performance goals may also be referred to as needs, particularly those related to better joint function, movement restoration, cardiovascular wellness, and overall health. Often clients do not recognize these needs or underestimate their importance, so they have not yet become goals in their minds. This is why a comprehensive assessment process should precede exercise selection and program design. What a person needs for optimal fitness and wellness should be prioritized appropriately in relation to goals of any type.

Aesthetic-Based Goals

Aesthetic-based goals relate to the physiological adaptations gained through exercise that affect appearance. Typically these goals involve desires for gains in muscle hypertrophy or muscle size as well as a decrease in body fat. However, changes in posture, which would often be categorized as a performance goal, will also dramatically affect appearance. The pursuit of aesthetic goals dominated the thought processes of the fitness industry for many years and has greatly influenced all aspects of resistance training such that magazines, instructional books, videos, certification courses, and even the design of resistance training equipment all were biased toward building bigger muscles.

In recent years throughout the fitness industry, there has been a wide swing toward focusing more on training for enhanced performance. This shift has again influenced literature, education, and equipment manufacturers—so much so that many fitness professionals are now completely negating the aesthetic benefits that are possible through resistance training and still most often desired by consumers at some level. Remember that most people will have a mix of both performance and aesthetic goals. This fact places you in a precarious position at times because you must select exercises, group them into programs, and use appropriate techniques to address all the needs and accomplish the primary goals of the client. This chapter should help you in this endeavor.

Targeting Desired Movements

The human body is capable of infinite combinations of movement patterns performed in a variety of postures and positions. Therefore exercise selection should consider the body's natural movement abilities and limits regardless of the training goal. Based on the theories of generalized movement patterns and study of human motor learning development, exercise movements can be split into two basic categories: general movement patterns and specific movement patterns. A resistance training program will likely contain some of both regardless of whether it is based on improvements in performance or aesthetics.

General Movement Patterns

General movement patterns (GMPs) are movements that maximize the use of the designed lever systems and relative biomechanical strengths to most efficiently interact within our natural environment. From birth, GMPs develop as humans develop control over their bodies; GMPs are typically established by the age of two years. However, as the body continues to age there is a tendency for increased joint wear, joint damage, faulty postural adaptations, and development of muscular imbalances that begin to deteriorate optimal movement abilities and induce compensation. Compensation eventually further deteriorates joint function to the point where GMPs are extremely limited and daily activity and quality of life are drastically reduced. Therefore maintenance or restoration of general movement pattern ability should be a performance goal at some level for most everyone's fitness program. Figure 5.1 illustrates the GMPs.

Motor learning and body control begin in the spine as infants start to develop the abilities to flex, extend, and eventually rotate the trunk before gaining much control over the arms and legs. Later, infants demonstrate the ability to operate arms and control hands, and they can perform basic pushing and pulling movements. Then, combining spinal and upper-body control with hip and leg movements, babies learn to crawl. Shortly after, they begin to push or pull themselves up and incorporate squat patterns as they learn to stand. From there, children progress from standing to walking as they attempt to master gait patterns.

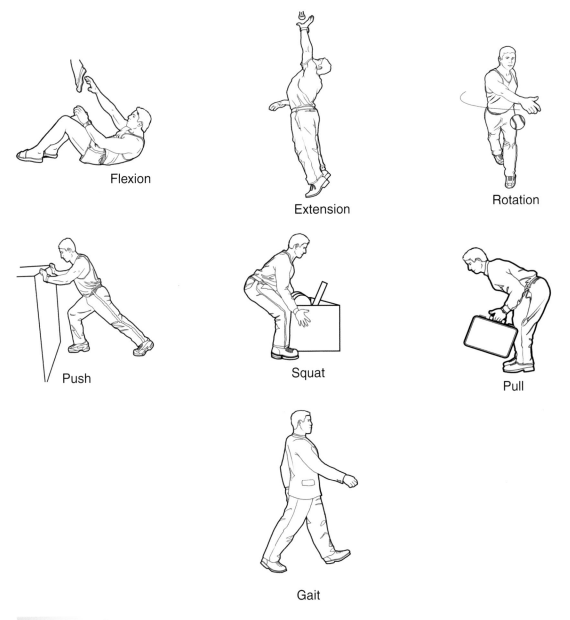

Flexion

Extension

Rotation

Push

Squat

Pull

Gait

Figure 5.1 General movement patterns.

Through biomechanical study and research of motor learning related to this process, we can identify seven distinct general movement patterns that enable humans to move and work on this planet. It is logical to assume that an effective resistance training program would include these movement patterns. Some of this theory was also adopted from studies by human performance specialist Paul Check, who has developed a training and rehabilitation system that he calls primal pattern movement. The following are the seven general movement patterns:

1. Spinal flexion
2. Spinal extension
3. Spinal rotation
4. Pushing patterns
5. Pulling patterns
6. Squat patterns
7. Gait patterns

Spinal Flexion

Of all spinal movements, forward flexion has the largest degree of available movement. This design allows humans to move and work with the environment directly in front, where the eyes, nose, and mouth are also located for efficient interaction between movement and senses. Muscle action for spinal flexion is performed by the abdominals and obliques. However, because gravity greatly assists with spinal flexion in standing and seated positions, humans rarely have high demands for abdominal and oblique work during typical life activities. These muscles are used more often for eccentric and isometric actions to resist external forces attempting to extend or rotate the spine. Therefore it makes sense to include exercises that train the abdominals eccentrically and isometrically in a resistance training program.

The spine does not flex as easily in every region. Because of the natural kyphotic, or preflexed, position of the thoracic spine, the mid back typically flexes at the greatest degree and with the least resistance. Conversely, because of the natural lordotic, or preextended, design of the spine in the lumbar and cervical regions (lower back and neck area, respectively), these sections are often the most difficult to flex. Over time, further decreased lumbar and cervical flexion leads to tissue restrictions and pain in the lower back and neck. Therefore exercise movements that target lumbar and cervical flexion should be included in a resistance training program, perhaps more than those movements that promote thoracic flexion, such as crunches. Figure 5.2 shows exercise selections targeting cervical flexion, thoracic flexion, and lumbar flexion.

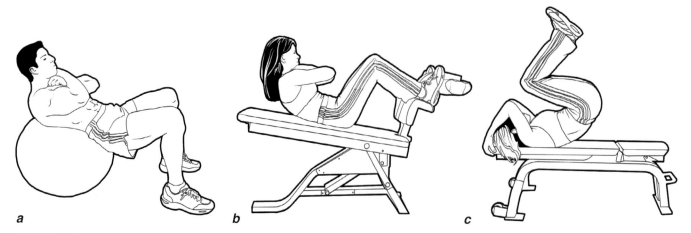

a *b* *c*

Figure 5.2 Exercise selections targeting *(a)* cervical flexion, *(b)* thoracic flexion, and *(c)* lumbar flexion.

Spinal Extension

Extension of the spine is naturally limited by design, particularly in the thoracic portion, which is the largest section of the spine. This limitation can also be considered an advantage when it comes to resisting extension forces attempting to bend the spine backward. However, the natural preflexed design of the thoracic spine makes it susceptible to developing forward postural deviations and posterior muscular weakness that result in reduced movements into extension and limited rotation. Therefore exercises that strengthen active thoracic extension (free from lumbar or cervical hyperextension) are important to include in a resistance training program for maintenance of general movement pattern ability. Also movements that incorporate hip extension with the spine stabilized in an optimal posture would be wise selections for maintaining a healthy spine. Figure 5.3, *a* and *b*, compares static thoracic extension with dynamic thoracic extension.

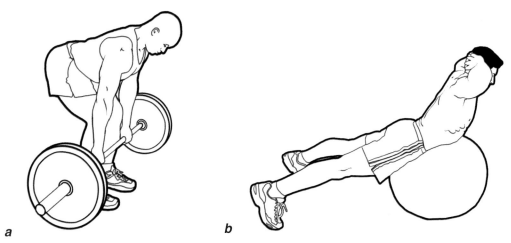

a *b*

Figure 5.3 Compare *(a)* static thoracic extension with *(b)* dynamic thoracic extension.

Spinal Rotation

Varying degrees of spinal rotation are integrated in all types of daily life activities. Therefore, the trunk is a critical component of all gait motion. However, exercises involving resisted spinal rotation and ballistic spinal rotation are often the highest-risk movements that can be selected. This is because a safe degree of rotation at any one vertebral joint is limited. There are 26 possible articulation points for spinal rotation; each possesses a varying degree of optimal movement ability that collectively contributes to the overall amount of spinal rotation. The rotation ability of the spine is extremely limited in the lumbar section but immediately increases in the thoracic section and opens up even more in the cervical section. Because spinal mechanics operate as a linked kinetic chain, any limitation in one section will encourage compensation and increased movement in the other sections. This compensatory movement begins to degenerate vertebral disks and stresses muscles and connective tissue, which eventually results in more limited movement at certain sections and accompanying compensation at others.

In short, optimal rotation of the spine is a complicated biomechanical process involving numerous musculoskeletal and neuromuscular components, so it must be trained cautiously. Limited spinal rotation should first be assessed by a trained practitioner because most conditions cannot be corrected simply through performance of rotational exercises. In fact, aggressive rotational exercises will often only induce further compensation and promote faster degeneration of the discs and connective tissues. Selection of exercises involving controlled and unloaded trunk rotation as well as exercises that stabilize against trunk rotation should precede selection of exercises involving actual resisted trunk rotation. Figure 5.4, *a, b, c,* compares these three options.

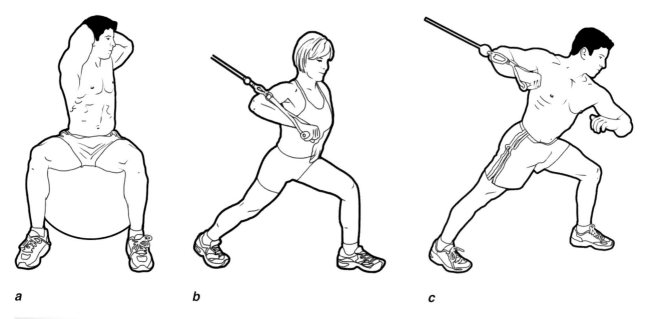

a　　　　　　　　　　　*b*　　　　　　　　　　　*c*

Figure 5.4　Compare *(a)* unresisted spinal rotation, *(b)* stabilized spinal rotation, and *(c)* resisted spinal rotation.

Pushing Patterns

The production of any movement is the result of muscles pulling on the skeletal levers of the body; therefore all muscles pull and there are technically no pushing muscles. To create a push pattern, you must combine two or more muscle pulls and associated joint motions that collectively produce a pushing force that can be applied against the ground or an object. Lower-body pushing patterns are classified as either squat movements or gait movements, both of which are covered in this chapter.

Upper-body pushing patterns directly involve varying degrees and positions of scapular, shoulder, elbow, and wrist movement. However, you should also consider stabilization requirements of the trunk and lower body when selecting pushing exercises. Because human movement is described in a three-plane system, we typically respond with exercise movements that are contained within one of these three planes. When selecting exercises, include movements in all three planes and consider exercise movements that are in between planes or even across more than one plane when appropriate. Single-arm pushing patterns and presses with offset loads (which places different weight loads in each arm) provide for various stabilization demands and can be used to target specific muscle synergies and subsystems. Figure 5.5, *a*, *b*, and *c*, shows examples of various pushing patterns performed in the three defined planes of motion.

Pulling Patterns

Pulling patterns are movements that incorporate two or more joint movements to produce a combined force that either pulls objects toward the body or pulls the body toward the object. Both are a similar action but are determined by the object's mass and stability rather than the mass and stability of the body. Pulling patterns involve varying degrees of scapular, shoulder, elbow, and wrist motion. Because humans are rarely required to do much climbing or pulling in today's life demands, it is important to include a variety of pulling movements in most any fitness program.

Pulling patterns target the back and postural muscles of the trunk but also can challenge the lower body depending on the exercises selected. Pulling patterns, as with the pushing patterns discussed previously, are typically presented as occurring in one of the three planes of movement. Pulling in all three as well as in between planes would also be advisable. Unilateral

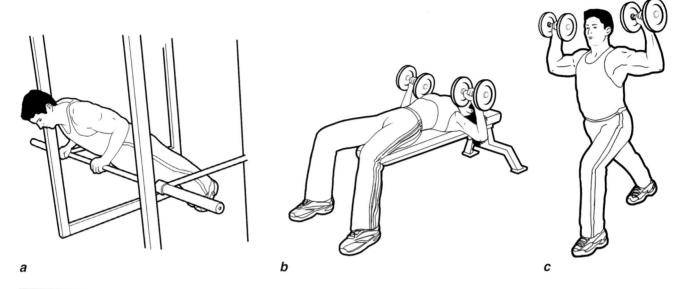

a   b   c

Figure 5.5 Pushing patterns *(a)* on the median plane, *(b)* on the horizontal plane, and *(c)* on the frontal plane.

(single-arm) pulling will also present different stabilization demands on the body and apply additional rotational forces to the spine, which require additional core and trunk muscle action. Figure 5.6, *a*, *b*, and *c*, shows examples of different pulling movements occurring in the three defined planes, each of which would also be used for accomplishing various goals or addressing various needs.

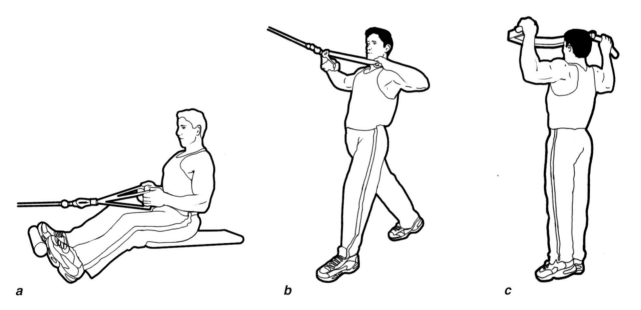

a   b   c

Figure 5.6 Pulling movements *(a)* of the median plane, *(b)* of the horizontal plane, and *(c)* of the frontal plane.

Squat Patterns

Squat patterns are some of the most basic and functional movements humans can use for accomplishing numerous daily tasks. Sitting or rising from a chair, picking up or setting down a box, and squatting and holding the position for a prolonged period in order to organize a drawer are all common examples of a squat pattern. Yet squats are often avoided or even purposefully restricted from an exercise program because of perceived risk. The squat itself is rarely a high-risk movement for most people, even those with back or knee problems. The real risk with the squat is usually associated with the technique a person uses when learning it or the manner and amount in which it is loaded.

The specific elements of technique used, such as the alignment, positioning, range of motion, stabilization, and tempo, are often the determining factor in the relative risk of the movement. As squat patterns in life are varied, so are the squat patterns in an exercise program. Load placement and amounts should also be varied accordingly. Figure 5.7, *a, b, c,* shows optional squat exercises that can help a person accomplish various goals or address different needs.

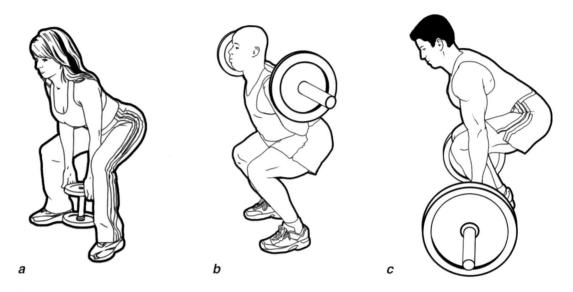

a   b   c

Figure 5.7   Squat exercises: *(a)* dumbbell wide squat, *(b)* barbell squat, and *(c)* barbell narrow squat.

Gait Patterns

Gait is the manner in which a person moves the body across the surface of the environment. Gait is typically pictured as walking but could be modified in a variety of ways, such as skipping, hopping, walking sideways, or even walking backward. A large variety of gait modifications exist to enable people to deal with different demands in life, such as direction changes, stride length and timing changes, and various level changes. Therefore there are also numerous choices of resistance training exercises for strengthening modified gait motions.

Movement speed, such as the transitions from walking to running and running to sprinting, are the most common variations of gait. As walking speed is increased, there is a need to modify the movement pattern to running, which calls for distinct timing and degrees of trunk, hip, knee, ankle, and arm movements. Body lean is slightly increased and foot strike tends to transition from a heel strike to a full-foot strike. As speed continues to increase from running to sprinting, another distinct modification to gait takes place, again requiring distinct timing and degrees of body and limb movements. Forward lean of the body increases and foot strike transitions to toe strike. Also as the inertia of the body is increased, less actual time is spent in contact with the ground.

Another common but often-overlooked gait variation occurs as the body needs to modify normal gait caused by a change in angle of movement or ground elevation as opposed to a change in speed of movement. Lunging up a hill or climbing a flight of stairs demands as much modification to normal gait as do running and sprinting. Figure 5.8, *a, b, c,* and *d,* demonstrate all these common gait variations.

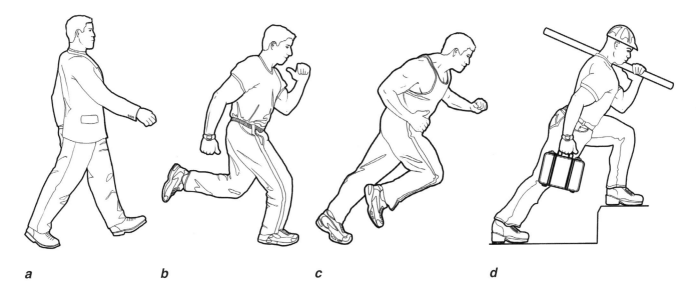

Figure 5.8 Gait variations: *(a)* walking, *(b)* running, *(c)* sprinting, and *(d)* lunging.

Certain joint weaknesses and muscular imbalances can induce compensation and alter optimal gait movement. Therefore, when attempting to improve a desired gait movement, simply practicing the movement does not typically increase performance; rather, it only reinforces compensation. Desired gait improvements can often occur through carefully selected resistance training exercises that either target specific muscle weakness or strengthen related muscle synergies, or subsystems, needed for improved gait movement. Certain therapies may also be necessary for treating serious joint dysfunctions.

Specific Movement Patterns

Specific movement patterns are multijoint or individual-joint movements that may address certain needs and help a person achieve performance-based goals or certain aesthetic-based goals. Countless exercise selections and variations are available. The specific movement patterns in this book represent only a small sample of the options available and address some of the most common performance- and aesthetic-based goals.

Targeting Desired Muscle Groups

Often, rather than selecting exercises according to the movement pattern they target, trainers may instead choose exercises according to the specific muscle group they target. Targeting muscles as opposed to movements is often considered to be typical for those focused on aesthetic goals. However, very often individual muscles or specific muscle groups or subsystems are targeted in order to correct muscular imbalances, improve posture, restore proper gait function, or attain some other performance-based goal. This demonstrates how exercise selection, whether done to target movement or target muscles, is not always correlated with only performance or aesthetic goals.

Muscular Synergies (Subsystems)

The control system rarely recruits individual muscles for any movement; rather, it recruits muscle synergies (subsystems). As all major body and limb movement is initiated through prior spinal movement or stability, the strengthening of the muscular synergies that control the trunk and pelvis are often considered a priority in a resistance training program. Five common muscle synergies have been presented by several experts as critical components for controlling movement and providing stability of the trunk and pelvis: the inner unit (core), the deep longitudinal subsystem (DLS), the lateral subsystem (LS), the posterior oblique subsystem (POS), and the anterior oblique subsystem (AOS).

Inner Unit (Core)

Several authors have cited research that has clearly identified a local stabilizing system known as the inner unit, or core. This deep collection of abdominal, pelvic, and spinal musculature performs dual functions for both respiration and stabilization. The inner unit is uniquely designed to accomplish both tasks simultaneously, and is under separate neurological control and can function independently from the outer and larger trunk muscles. The inner unit provides for critical spinal intersegmental control and local spinal and pelvic stabilization. Conversely, the outer and larger trunk muscles such as the rectus abdominis, spinal erectors, obliques, and certain hip muscles work as global spinal stabilizers and provide the force needed for actual trunk movement. Some authors include all these muscles as part of the core, but in this book these muscles are listed separately as trunk, or hip, muscles.

The core is composed of superior, inferior, anterior, and posterior muscles that enclose the contents of the abdominal cavity, or viscera. The core muscles provide intra-abdominal pressure to stabilize the spine while still performing respiratory functions. The primary muscles of the core are the diaphragm, the pelvic floor muscles, the transverse abdominis, and deep spinal muscles collectively known as the transversospinalis group. However, deep spinal muscles, such as the posterior fibers of the internal obliques, the quadratus lumborum, and the psoas muscles, all contribute to pelvic lumbar stability and are also considered by some authors as part of the core.

The transverse abdominis muscles as well as other core and trunk muscles attach to the spine through a large, broad, flattened tendon called the thoracolumbar aponeurosis, which is also known as the thoracolumbar fascia. The thoracolumbar aponeurosis is a network of noncontractile tendonlike tissue laid out in anterior, middle, and posterior layers. It plays a vital role in spinal stabilization and provides a critical force transference mechanism for the various muscular subsystems of the body. It also is a critical component of the core.

The core is involved not only in stabilization but also in respiration. These two seemingly opposing roles are actually harmonious actions consistent with the core's designed function. The breathing method presented in chapter 4 is based on the core's dual roles of assisting with respiration while providing local stabilization of the spine. The following sections describe how the core muscles work synergistically during the inhalation and exhalation phases of respiration.

Inhalation The diaphragm is a dome-shaped muscle that originates along the lower ribs and inserts along the anterior surfaces on the lower thoracic and lumbar spine. If unrestricted, the diaphragm initiates inhalation and helps the lungs to draw in air and expand the thoracic cavity by creating a downward push on the contents of the abdominal cavity (viscera) as pictured in figure 5.9. This downward force increases intra-abdominal pressure and pushes the viscera down against the bowl of the pelvis. This in turn signals a cocontraction of the pelvic floor muscles, which assists with stabilization of the pelvic and sacral joints. The viscera also press backward, which signals a cocontraction of the multifidi and assisting transversospinalis muscles, which assist to stabilize the lower and middle levels of the spine. The increased intra-abdominal pressure also begins to cause the viscera to distend forward, creating passive tension in the transverse abdominis and a tightening of the thoracolumbar fascia, which further stabilizes the pelvis and stiffens the spine.

A concert of spinal and costal muscles completes inhalation by expanding and slightly elevating the rib cage. This action further extends the thoracic spine and results in an increased and straightened posture. At full inhalation both the abdominal and thoracic cavities are pressurized, and support for optimal stabilization is provided from the inside out. At this point, simply holding the breath and tightening abdominal muscles create a Valsalva maneuver and provides for maximal stability of the spine. The Valsalva maneuver is a natural protective mechanism and is sometimes initiated automatically when balance or spinal stability is suddenly challenged. However, longer-term use of the Valsalva maneuver for even several seconds can quickly increase blood pressure and reduce oxygen flow, which pose certain risks and is not recommended.

Exhalation The greater challenge for spinal and postural stabilization occurs during exhalation as pressure is being lost from both the abdominal and thoracic cavities. However, through a contraction of the transverse abdominis, this pressure loss is minimized and core activation is increased to assist with continued stabilization. The contraction of the transverse abdominis (as pictured in figure 5.10), creates a drawing in of the viscera (much like the tightening of a wide belt) and presses the viscera back, down, and upward, which maintains greater levels of intra-abdominal and intrathoracic pressure. This pressure, coupled with cocontractions of the pelvic floor muscles, multifidi, deep erector muscles, posterior fibers of the internal oblique, and a reciprocal relaxation of the diaphragm, helps to maintain spinal and pelvic stabilization while assisting with exhalation.

Control of intra-abdominal pressure is believed by some to be an automated action for the lower levels of stabilization needed for most daily activities. Therefore it is believed to require no voluntary core activation and no specified breathing method. However, efficient core function can become inhibited through injury, surgery, immune system stress, disease, or perhaps practice of faulty exercise and breathing techniques. Also consider that resistance training frequently challenges the body by using additional load and requires more repetitive movements than typically encountered in most daily activities. Both facts support the reasoning for incorporating specific core activation and breathing methods as elements of technique.

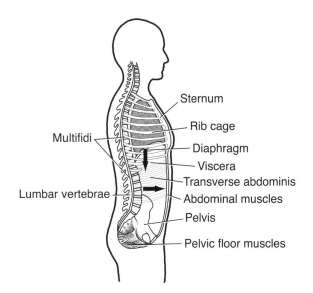

Figure 5.9 Inhalation.

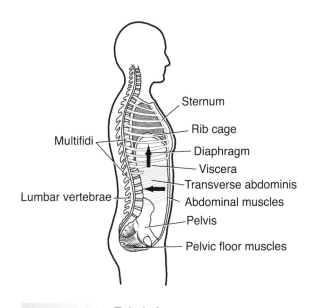

Figure 5.10 Exhalation.

Deep Longitudinal Subsystem

The deep longitudinal subsystem (DLS) helps to stabilize the body from ankle to head. It also provides for reciprocal force transmission from the ground to the trunk and back down. The DLS includes the tibialis anterior, peroneus longus, biceps femoris, sacrotuberous ligament, erector spinae, and thoracolumbar fascia. The dominant roles of the DLS take place during the stance phase of gait as it works to stabilize the ankle, decelerate forward leg movement, stabilize the spine, and control kinetic energy resulting from the heel striking the ground.

As the leg moves forward during the swing phase when walking or running, the hamstring muscles activate just enough to decelerate the forward leg movement or hip flexion and knee extension. The activation of the biceps femoris increases tension in the sacrotuberous ligament, which transfers force across the sacrum, which stabilizes the sacroiliac (SI) joint of the pelvis and allows for force transference up through the erector spinae to help stabilize the trunk. The tightening of the biceps femoris also causes tension through the peroneus longus, which works in concert with the anterior tibialis to stabilize the ankle in preparation for the heel to strike the ground. Upon heel strike, the ankle, hip, and spine are stabilized and resulting ground forces are captured in the thoracolumbar fascia and transferred to the posterior oblique system for the subsequent propulsion phase of gait, as pictured in figure 5.11.

Lateral Subsystem

The lateral subsystem (LS) works with the DLS in stabilizing impact during the stance phase of gait but does so in the frontal plane. It is composed of the hip abductor musculature (gluteus medius, gluteus minimus, tensor fasciae latae) and the contralateral, or opposite side, trunk lateral flexors (quadratus lumborum, internal obliques), with some assisting control from the ipsilateral, or same side, hip adductors. Upon heel strike, the ipsilateral hip abductors work in unison with the contralateral lateral trunk musculature to dynamically stabilize the pelvis, control center of gravity, and provide a level base of support for the spine. The lateral flexors of the spine assist with a slight lateral tilt of the pelvis, or hip hike, to allow for opposite-side leg lift, which will assist with the subsequent swing phase and actions of the anterior oblique subsystem.

Gait movements that involve accelerated side-to-side motion, such as in sports like football, speed skating, or tennis, rely heavily on a strong and well-synchronized lateral subsystem. In figure 5.12 the LS and its actions are pictured during a specific gait movement that would further challenge this subsystem.

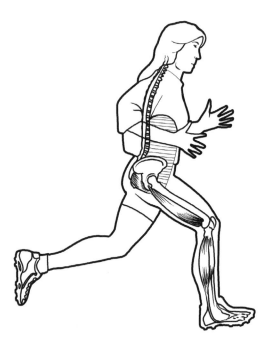

Figure 5.11 The deep longitudinal subsystem.

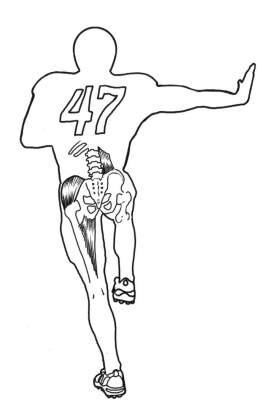

Figure 5.12 The lateral subsystem.

Posterior Oblique Subsystem

The posterior oblique subsystem (POS) is composed primarily of the latissimus dorsi and the contralateral, or opposite side, gluteus maximus. The POS works synergistically with the DLS through transference of kinetic energy across their shared attachments into the thoracolumbar fascia. The POS is dominant in the propulsion phase of gait and also decelerates limb movements during the swing phase. The POS is also important in rotational actions such as swinging an implement and throwing a ball. It cocks the body for initiation of any ballistic rotational movement and then decelerates that same motion.

During the swing phase of gait, the ipsilateral gluteus maximus of the POS assists the hamstrings in decelerating hip flexion and forward leg motion while the contralateral latissimus dorsi works to decelerate trunk rotation and swing of the arm. There is a parallel alignment of the muscle fibers of the gluteus maximus and the contralateral latissimus dorsi. They run perpendicular to the sacroiliac joint, which helps to stabilize the pelvis during the impact of heel strike and prepares the entire lumbar–pelvic region for propulsion.

The thoracolumbar fascia then transfers stored kinetic energy to the POS, which in turn accelerates the respective limbs and propels the body forward. The timing of the cocontraction of the POS produces tension that is again transferred to the thoracolumbar fascia. This tension assists with continued pelvic and lumbar stabilization and can also be stored for use in the subsequent phases of gait, which reduces the metabolic cost of gait. Figure 5.13 depicts the POS during gait motion.

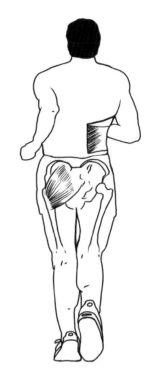

Figure 5.13 The posterior oblique subsystem.

Anterior Oblique Subsystem

The anterior oblique subsystem (AOS) works similarly to the POS but from an anterior orientation. The AOS is composed primarily of the adductors of the hip with their ipsilateral internal obliques and contralateral external obliques. The AOS is dominant for the swing phase of gait but is also instrumental in accelerating rotational movements such as when throwing objects or swinging implements.

The hip adductors work with the contralateral obliques through the parallel alignment of their fibers and the proximity of attachment at the pubis, which facilitate force transference and communication between the two muscle groups. The muscles of the AOS work synergistically to stabilize the body on top of the stance leg while rotating the pelvis for the swing phase of gait. The AOS also works with the POS to help with optimal positioning of the pelvis and leg for impact from the succeeding heel strike. The AOS is depicted in figure 5.14 during the swing phase of gait.

In addition to these deep subsystems of the trunk, you should consider other common muscle synergies when selecting resistance exercises. These muscle synergies correspond directly to the movements used most in daily life and are associated with the seven general movement patterns presented in this chapter. Therefore, by basing your exercise selection on targeting both movements and muscle groups involved in flexing, extending, and rotating the spine as well as pushing, pulling, squatting, and those that strengthen gait movement, you should have a good foundation on which to build training routines and design effective exercise programs.

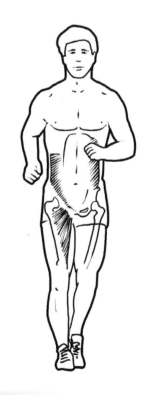

Figure 5.14 The anterior oblique subsystem.

Isolation of Specific Muscles

Selecting exercises for isolating specific muscles is not reserved for bodybuilders or those training for primarily cosmetic results. Exercises selected for their ability to produce hypertrophy of an isolated muscle are more than likely an aesthetically driven decision. Exercises that isolate chest, shoulders, arms, quads, hamstrings, and calves for the sole purpose of increasing the size of these muscles is still rather common and can be found in numerous books, magazines, and DVDs. However, isolating specific muscles for strengthening is often necessary for correction of muscular imbalances and restoration of efficient joint mechanics, which are totally performance-based selections. These exercises often include isolated strengthening of the rotator cuff, shoulder, wrist, hip, knee, and ankle musculatures. These movements are not as common in fitness resources but often appear in rehabilitation and physical therapy books.

This text focuses primarily on general movement patterns and the targeting of muscle synergies, so it does not provide large amounts of isolated joint movement exercises. However, a balanced sampling has been included in order to demonstrate the differences in exercise selection available for addressing performance needs or striving to accomplish aesthetic goals.

Determining Risks Versus Benefits of Selection

For a movement of any joint to take place, a force and a transference of force need to occur. As any joint receives and transfers forces through the body and to the environment, there is always a stress and inherent risk of damage to the joint. However, because joint movement is essential for joint health, you must move your body in order to maintain or improve its function. Therefore, for any resistance training exercise, there is always a ratio of risk to perceived benefit. You must understand benefits are often only perceived, whereas risks are always real. Therefore you must become more cognitive of all the risks involved in any exercise selection, because the risks are present whether you know it or not.

You can assess any movement for its potential benefits and inherent risks. You must eventually apply this information to each person's set of conditions and abilities in order to determine relative benefits or risks associated with an exercise. To fully understand the potential risk of any exercise, you would have to present a tremendous amount of information associated with the physics of the movement itself, in-depth structural analysis of each involved joint, and all the associated physiological and biomechanical issues. Then, to compare potential risk with the potential benefits, you would have to present an equal amount of information concerning the person's unique structure, genetics, and abilities for stress adaptation.

The information in chapter 1 provides you with critical information on the structures and functions of the human body in order to help you assess risk and recognize the potential benefits offered from any resistance exercise. Also, you should be assured that years of research and practical experience were applied in the selection of exercises and techniques for this book. Many exercises that are considered too high risk relative to potential benefits were intentionally omitted. However, that does not mean that no other safe or efficient exercises are available, nor should you assume that every exercise presented is appropriate for achieving the goals of every person. However, the exercise selections combined with the associated suggestions for exercise technique should prove effective and safe for most healthy people that you may train.

Resistance Exercise Program Design

If you ask almost any fitness enthusiast or even most fitness professionals about what makes up a resistance program, you will probably get a similar response. A resistance training program is typically viewed as a collection of selected exercises grouped together for the purpose of accomplishing a person's goals. Although this sounds like a logical answer, it is actually a definition of a routine rather than a program. It is this same simplistic approach to programming that often leads to only minimal progress, failure to reach a goal, and programs that often completely ignore the person's needs. This chapter, though only a summary of all that could be presented on this topic, should help you understand the primary concepts involved in resistance exercise programming and help you develop the thought process necessary for organizing your exercise selections to build effective routines and design effective training programs for your clients and athletes. Programming is a science, but it is also an art to those who practice and provide fitness programs professionally. By becoming well acquainted with the information provided in this chapter, you should also be able to better develop your own skills in program design for yourself and those you may serve.

Routines Versus Programs

According to the strict definitions of the words, there are differences between a routine and a program. Yet in fitness, these terms are often used interchangeably. Let's look at the definitions of these two words before we discuss the meanings and differences from a fitness perspective.

routine—A ritual; a series of actions or behaviors performed on a regular basis; repetitive practice.

This is exactly how many people approach their fitness programs and precisely why their progress is limited. To believe that continued progress can be achieved by simply performing a collection of movement patterns on a repetitive, or routine, basis would be contrary to all we have come to know about the human body. We know that muscles have the ability to adapt to certain stimuli. But without progressive stimuli, there cannot be progressive adaptation. All exercises are specific movement patterns that provide only a limited and specific set of stimuli. Once that set of stimuli has been learned and adapted to, not much more information can be obtained until the movement has been modified in some manner. This means that without new input, new adaptations are unlikely, which may be sufficient for maintenance but does not offer much opportunity for progression.

program—A specific system of instructions; to provide a detailed set of instructions for achieving a specific purpose; a purposeful plan of action.

These definitions most often refer to how programs are used by a computer. Coincidentally, many experts on motor learning compared the functions of the control (sensorimotor) system to a very advanced computer system. The control system processes all stimuli supplied by any exercise movement, compares the information to original instructions, attempts to perfect the movement, then stores the movement for future recall. Meanwhile, the active and passive systems attempt to adapt physiologically to the stresses and demands of the exercise in order to develop muscles and strengthen joints. These adaptations can lead to enhancement of biomotor abilities such as strength, endurance, mobility, stability, speed, power, and agility. As a by-product of these processes, muscles may also increase in size (hypertrophy), and body fat reduction may occur, which will alter the composition and change the body's appearance. However, all adaptations depend on the stimuli provided by the specific exercises and techniques selected and organized into the program. Therefore, better definitions for routines and programs relative to exercise can be derived and stated as follows:

routine—A collection of carefully selected exercise movements performed with specific techniques for a specified period.

program—A planned series of routines that are systematically varied in a purposeful and specific manner in order to achieve periodic goals and address identified needs.

This chapter ties together all information provided in earlier chapters in order to help you group selected exercises into realistic yet challenging routines and then organize and vary the routines to create short-term, medium-term, and long-term (periodized) programs.

Variables of Resistance Training

Once you have selected an exercise movement, you have many choices for varying that exercise. Think of the almost infinite number of ways you could vary any resistance exercise, such as alignment, positioning, stabilization strategies, path, range or speed of motion, amount of resistance applied, frequency of the exercise, order of the exercise in a routine, and amount of rest between exercises. A well-designed program consists of planned cycles broken down into specific phases that will guide how each variable of every exercise can be manipulated. Variables of resistance training may be divided into five general categories:

1. Technique
2. Intensity
3. Volume
4. Recovery
5. Sequence

Chapter 4 of this book provides detailed information on all elements of efficient and safe technique. Therefore, this chapter won't cover these concepts again, other than to reiterate that technique is always an option that you should consider before beginning an exercise. Technique is the most important variable for any resistance training exercise and will largely determine the success or failure of the entire program.

Intensity

Next to technique, intensity is possibly the most influential variable a person can manipulate for any exercise. In fact, intensity and technique are interdependent. Certain technique options will limit or support the amount of intensity, just as intensity levels can greatly influence most every element of technique. Therefore, I choose to use only intensity loads that allow for performance of the exercise within the alignment, positioning, motion, stabilization, tempo, and sometimes even the breathing method desired. However, that does not mean that intensity is kept low; rather, it is matched appropriately with the exercise and technique options selected.

Intensity is the level of effort produced compared to the maximal effort possible. In resistance training, intensity is measured relative to the load, or amount of resistance, used. Intensity levels largely determine the specific type of adaptations the body attempts to achieve and also directly affect all other exercise variables. Intensity is often related to the principle of progressive overload, which states that sufficient intensity and duration must be applied to overload the muscles' present levels of adaptation in order to improve strength or endurance. Intensity loads are often expressed as a percentage of a one-repetition maximum effort (or percent of 1RM). However, because actually testing a person's maximal effort for a single repetition on any exercise would constitute a high risk, it is better to simply pick the weight that is appropriate for performance of the movement for the approximate desired duration and within the technique selected. When selecting a weight load for a client or athlete on a new exercise, always start with low levels or possibly even no added resistance in order for the client to first learn the movement pattern and begin practicing technique.

Intensity and Volume

The relationship of intensity to volume is probably the most critical to understand because several components of volume should be adjusted as intensity is changed. Overall, the common belief is that there should be an inverse relationship between intensity and volume. The debate is in how much volume should be decreased relative to an increase in intensity. The following sections provide some direction in adjusting the reps, tempos, and sets relative to adjustments in intensity.

Intensity and Repetitions   One component of volume that is relatively easy to adjust in relation to changes in intensity is the number of repetitions performed. This relationship is automatically regulated by the person's current neuromuscular abilities. As intensity increases, the repetitions naturally decrease, leading to the desired objective of decreased total volume. The opposite is also true—if intensity is decreased, then more repetitions are possible, which may result in increases in total volume. The relationship of intensity to repetitions should be acknowledged but should not dictate actual increases or decreases in total volume. This decision should be predetermined by the program and accounted for in the assignment of all other components of volume for each phase of each cycle. Intensity-to-volume relationships can easily be controlled with even minimal amounts of planning, because every other component of volume is a choice that is not directly determined by the intensity.

Intensity and Tempo   Intensity should influence tempo. The natural effect of greater resistance is that it will move faster as it is lowered and move slower as it is raised because heavier loads are more difficult to decelerate and accelerate. However, tempo can have a dramatic effect on the specific type of strength adaptations that are achieved. Therefore, assignment of specific repetition speeds should be predetermined by the program rather than dictated by the intensity loads. That said, intensity will influence tempo, particularly as intensity levels are increased. Since it is proportionally more difficult to control heavier loads, tempo should generally be slowed when intensity is increased. This recommendation does not apply, however, to power-related movements, such as cleans and snatches. These types of movements incorporate techniques that rely on higher speeds of movement to accelerate loads toward their ending positions. These movements are often performed with relatively less load than is squatted, pressed, and pulled by the same person in other exercises. Cleans, snatches and similar plyometric type movements also involve higher levels of risk, particularly for those people who have not yet mastered the associated techniques or who have existing structural or neuromuscular problems. The greatest risk is typically not in the acceleration of the weight load or object, but rather during the deceleration or lowering of the weight. Here again, practice with proper technique is vital for reducing the risk of injury.

Intensity and Sets   The number of sets performed is always a choice, one that is often given little thought. A well-established, yet rarely applied, training principle addresses this issue. This principle simply states that as intensity increases and repetitions decrease, the number of sets should be increased if certain levels of volume are important to maintain. That is particularly true for anyone who desires muscle growth (hypertrophy). Hypertrophy is the increase in muscle size that accompanies tissue adaptations to stress created from the combination of intensity and volume of resistance training. If sets are not added to offset the reduction of repetitions in response to higher-intensity loads, the resulting decrease in total volume often makes it difficult to gain or even maintain desired levels of hypertrophy.

Intensity, Duration, and Frequency

The general recommendation is to maintain an inverse relationship between intensity on one hand and duration and frequency on the other. The duration of an individual set is obviously immediately affected inversely by intensity changes as the time under tension will drop as load increases. Duration of a routine, however, is determined by the total volume of all exercises performed in that session, which may also be advisable to adjust. Frequency adjustments are another choice that should be considered relevant to changes in intensity. Because more recovery time is typically recommended as intensity is increased, it might be wise for some people to decrease the frequency of their workout sessions. This may not fit in with some people's other goals, or it may not be realistic. Therefore, you can design the program to focus on a different area of the body in each session during phases in which you're using higher intensity levels in order to allow for ample recovery yet stay on the current schedule. This planned approach will reduce the frequency of the stimulus for each area of the body without changing the frequency of the actual training sessions.

Intensity and Exercise Selections   Since any resistance exercise emphasizes the use of certain muscle groups, whether intentionally or unintentionally, most exercises can be classified by the muscles they target. Therefore, you should consider the total amount of exercises selected per body part in a given routine when making adjustments to intensity and volume. When increasing intensity, decreasing reps, adding sets, and using slower tempos, it is also logical to reduce the number of exercises per body part. This not only helps to maintain proper ratios of volume and intensity but also provides for the extra recovery needed when working with heavier loads. It can also allow for adherence to preplanned duration and frequency changes.

It is clear that there is much to consider when determining the changes in volume that should accompany changes in intensity. People who carry on routines for too long with intensity–volume relationships that are too high can experience overtraining, fatigue, decreases in performance, impaired health, and increased risk of injury. Conversely, routines that contain intensity–volume relationships that are too low not only lack sufficient work for muscle hypertrophy but also may not provide enough stimulation for significant improvements in strength. The routines also may not elicit the beneficial hormonal responses conducive for increased metabolic activity and fat loss. Table 6.1 depicts all the various intensity–volume relationships and the changes in each component of volume that can be adjusted in relation to increases in intensity. This chart should help you understand these relationships so you can design more effective resistance training programs.

TABLE 6.1 Volume and Intensity Relationships

Training goals	Intensity	Repetitions	Sets	Sub-total 1	Tempo assignment	Sub-total 2	Exercise/ muscle group	Initial volume	Rest between sets
Endurance	X	17	2	34 reps	2111 (5 sec)	170 sec	3	510 sec	30-60 sec
Hypertrophy	X+Y	10	3	30 reps	3121 (7 sec)	210 sec	2	420 sec	60-240 sec
Strength	X+Y+Z	5	5	25 reps	4122 (9 sec)	225 sec	1	225 sec	300+ sec

Intensity and Recovery

When intensity is increased, it not only stresses the joints and tissues of the passive and active systems, but it also stresses and drains the neural system. It is believed that nerve cells take at least five times as long as muscle cells to recover. In certain high-intensity training phases, rest intervals of up to eight minutes between sets are not uncommon. This allows for more complete neural recovery as well as metabolic recovery. As seen in table 6.1, you should allow more planned recovery time when using higher-intensity loads. However, rest periods between sets do not need to be absolute in most phases of training. Often an active recovery, such as performing supersets with movement patterns that are opposite or unrelated to the previous movement and target different muscle groups, is an option to consider between sets. This allows for adequate recovery of the specific motor units previously recruited, but it also supplies more opportunity for increased overall work. This is a logical choice in certain phases because usually other movement patterns and muscle groups also need to be trained in order to accomplish overall training goals.

Intensity and Sequence

The intensity level of an exercise will also dictate its preferred placement in the sequence of the routine. The higher the intensity level, the more the neural demand, so the earlier in the routine it would logically be placed. However, certain biomechanical factors—such as the exercise's effect on stabilizers needed for subsequent movements or the priority of overall goals—may occasionally cause a change to this sequencing guideline. It is also reasonable to purposely spread intense exercises throughout the routine rather than place them all at the beginning. This would require a more consistent level of effort throughout the routine and would likely promote a more consistent hormonal response as well. In any case, always keep in mind that the later a high-intensity exercise is placed in the sequence of a routine, the worse the performance is likely to be.

Volume

Volume for a muscle is the total amount of time it is placed under tension. This can be broken down into initial volume (the total amount of time under tension for a given muscle during a single routine) and total volume. Initial volume (IV) is calculated by multiplying the number of repetitions by the number of sets, and then multiplying again by the time it takes to complete each repetition, which would be determined by the assigned tempo. Each movement that targets that area would also need to be considered for determining initial volume (IV = reps × sets × tempo × exercise per muscle group). Total volume can be calculated for a given phase, mesocycle, macrocycle, or weekly, monthly, or quarterly time periods simply by multiplying the initial volume of each routine by the frequency with which it was performed during the phase, cycle, or time period desired. Tracking volume is a simple matter of disciplined record keeping, which is more easily accomplished if the amounts of desired volume for each muscle group during each routine were previously planned and directed by the program. This preplanning and calculation help to provide for volumes that are consistent for the desired goals. However, because daily adjustments are often needed for any plan, the actual volume is more related to achieving results as opposed to the plan itself.

Repetitions

The amount of time a muscle is under tension will determine its adaptive response, making the amount of repetitions an important component of volume. In fact, the desired time under tension, and therefore the repetitions, should be used in selecting the intensity loads as opposed to letting the intensity dictate the repetitions. The repetitions combined with the prescribed tempo dictate the duration of any set, which determine the energy systems and muscle fiber types that will be trained and the neural-metabolic adaptations a person can expect from that set. Because neural-metabolic adaptations are a part of most people's goals (whether they know it or not), they should be planned. That is, all components of volume, including specific repetition ranges, should also be planned rather than random.

Greater neural and intramuscular adaptations are experienced with sets performed at higher intensities and with shorter times under tension. Low-repetition sets with higher intensities also require more use of the short-term energy system, or ATP-CP (adenosine triphosphate-creatine phosphate). This combination would also recruit more type IIb muscle fibers, which would be more appropriate for strength and power goals. Conversely, high-repetition sets performed with lighter loads work more into the aerobic (oxidative) energy system and require more activation of type IIc and type I muscle fibers. These muscle fibers and this energy system are ideal for use in activities requiring greater amounts of muscular endurance. Moderate-repetition sets with moderate-intensity loads require more contributions from the glycolytic or lactic acid energy systems and target the various type IIa fibers. This middle zone provides the stimulus for a blend of strength and endurance adaptations and is also associated with the greatest increases in muscle hypertrophy. For this reason, many resources recommend constant mid-range repetition and intensity combinations for development of hypertrophy. However, a program that periodically varies the repetitions (along with all other components of volume) and intensity tend to allow greater gains. Table 6.2 depicts the correlation of time under tension with the energy systems, muscle fiber types, and neural-metabolic adaptations.

By using this chart, you can determine the proper duration of any set for the desired training goals. Select the amount of resistance that will be challenging during the time under tension. Estimates of the number of repetitions performed that correspond to the targeted amount of time under tension are also given. When using these numbers, however, it is assumed that an average tempo of six seconds per repetition is used. More or fewer reps can be produced in the same time under tension by adjusting the tempo, but this should cause little change in neural-metabolic adaptations. However, different tempos may elicit different types of specific strength adaptations.

TABLE 6.2　Neural-Metabolic Continuum of Adaptation

Energy system (continuum)	Primary muscle fiber types stimulated	Time under tension	Neural-metabolic adaptation (continuum)	Specific training goals	Suggested recovery between sets
ATP-PC	IIB	1-10 secs (1-2 reps)*	Neural adaptation	Strength/power	5+ min
	IIaB IIAB IIAb	30-90 secs (6-15 reps)*		Strength-hypertrophy	
Glycolytic/lactic acid				Hypertrophy	
	IIA				1-4 min
	IIAC IIC	180+ secs (30+ reps)*	Metabolic adaptation	Hypertrophy-endurance	
Oxidative/aerobic					0-30 secs
	IC I			Endurance	

*Average tempo of 6 seconds

Tempo

Tempo is the specific speed of a given repetition. Tempo has a much more dramatic training effect than simply its contribution to volume. Tempo is also a part of technique and can have a definitive influence on the specific type of strength that will be developed. Mechanoreceptors known as muscle spindles are sensitive to the speed of muscle contraction. They relay detailed information on changes in the length and tension of the muscles to the appropriate level of the control system for processing. Once information on speed of contraction, speed of force production, and rate of acceleration is learned and stored in the control system, specific intramuscular adaptations can then be recalled and used for similar demands in appropriate situations. As presented in chapter 4, I prefer to assign tempo with the use of a four-digit number that represents the number of seconds for each phase and therefore dictates the precise movement speed throughout the repetition. The first digit represents the eccentric phase, the second the eccentric–isometric phase, the third the concentric phase, and the fourth the concentric–isometric phase.

Certain tempos are more suited for achieving specific types of strength gains, such as maximal strength, static strength, explosive strength, and starting (acceleration) strength needed for improved speed. For example, stability strength would benefit from slow, controlled tempos with pauses at critical points of the movement to develop stronger joint stability, such as a 2421 tempo. Gains in starting speed strength would require a tempo with pauses at the eccentric–isometric phase combined with a fast concentric phase of the repetition to teach the muscle to contract quickly from a set prelengthened position, such as a 2201 tempo. On the other hand, explosive strength would benefit most from a tempo that assigns a quick eccentric movement immediately followed by a quick concentric movement, with no pause in between in order to use the stretch reflex to increase power, such as a 1011 tempo. For general strength and hypertrophy goals, a controlled eccentric and concentric phase with slight pauses at the changeover points, such as a 2121 or a 3120, is recommended. Keep in mind that 0 simply implies that movement through this phase is done as fast as possible.

Sets

The number of sets performed is always an option, regardless of intensity levels or repetitions. Recommendations in current literature range from 1 to 12 sets depending on the goals. As previously discussed, there is good reason to plan an inverse relationship between the number of sets and the number of repetitions performed and a correlating relationship of sets with changes in intensity. This principle of increasing sets proportionally with an increase in intensity in order to maintain a certain level of overall volume can be altered for special cases when increased strength along with maintenance of or decrease in muscle hypertrophy are desired. This may be the case with a wrestler or a figure skater who wishes to get stronger but has no desire for increased muscle size. For these athletes, working with heavier loads and allowing the volume to decrease at a steeper rate may make sense. However, large and even moderate amounts of muscle hypertrophy are not as easy to achieve as some people fear and most likely will not happen by accident.

Overall body mass, muscle size, muscle type, gender, and current level of conditioning all influence the number of sets prescribed. Larger people tend to receive greater benefits from more sets than smaller people do. Larger muscles typically respond better to more sets than smaller muscles. Fast-twitch muscles develop better with more sets and heavier loads, whereas slow-twitch muscles respond more to fewer sets with lighter loads. The average male responds better to more sets than the average female does. More experienced and better conditioned people will tolerate and often need more sets and overall volume in order to experience progress. Conversely, beginners cannot recover from higher volumes of training and can often benefit from as little as one set. The training goals will also influence the choices of sets. Yet no matter the reasoning, the focus should always be on the quality of the sets rather than the quantity.

Duration

Duration is another component of volume that you should plan well when designing resistance exercise programs. Duration is a general term that could be used to describe almost any portion of volume, such as the duration of a single repetition or set; the duration of a routine or session; and the duration of a phase, cycle, or overall program. The duration of a repetition is the total tempo time and should be determined by the specific type of strength gains desired. Duration of a set is based on the neural-metabolic adaptations needed in order to achieve strength, hypertrophy, or endurance goals. The duration of a routine is based primarily on the total number of sets and the amount of recovery given between each set. This can vary and may be determined by the person's current condition or the time the person has available for training. Recommended duration of a routine or single session of resistance training is typically 30 to 60 minutes as glycogen stores will become depleted and hormonal responses may begin to wane. The duration of phases, cycles, and programs depends totally on the overall program design and is discussed later in this chapter.

Frequency

Frequency relates to how often an exercise, a routine, a phase, or a cycle is performed. The frequency of any exercise is dependent on several factors. A complex or new exercise must be performed often enough in order to learn, develop, and store the motor program. Often if exercise frequency is inconsistent, proper technique cannot be integrated and faulty motor programs are developed that can make it more difficult to correct than if starting from scratch. On the other hand, if frequency of the same exercise is too constant and of high volume, it can lead to pattern overload, which may lead to muscular imbalances, stress connective tissue, and cause increased wear of joint surfaces.

Frequency of a routine really depends on the person's schedule, lifestyle, priorities, and commitment to the fitness program. In a perfect setting you would set frequency of routines based on the training phase, current cycle, and the person's ability to recover. This means frequency would vary as planned throughout the year as part of the overall program design. However, because that is rarely the case, it is best to keep frequency aligned with whatever schedule the person can commit to at the time. For most people frequency will vary throughout the year because work, family, and other life demands all affect their ability to adhere as consistently as they hoped or planned. Therefore, I recommend setting the frequency before designing the program, because this may influence every other program variable more than any other single factor, starting with whether the routines will be full body or split.

Recovery

Recovery is an essential variable for performance of a set or the entire routine. It is influenced by intensity and should be closely correlated with initial and overall volume. Recovery is necessary for the adaptation process, and tissue repair may take 2 to 10 days after a single session, depending on the intensity, volume, muscle fiber type, and the conditioning of the person. All muscles recover at different rates; larger ones take longer than smaller ones and fast-twitch muscles take longer than slow-twitch muscles. Larger people may also take longer to recover than smaller people, depending on condition, experience with training, and genetics. Therefore, large people performing exercise routines that include high-intensity, low-rep training targeting larger fast-twitch muscles will probably need more recovery and less frequency than smaller people performing low-intensity, high-rep training that targets smaller, slow-twitch muscles. Remember that muscles can become stronger, gain endurance, or hypertrophy only on the days they rest.

Lack of recovery between workout routines leads to exhaustion and overtraining. Exhaustion is the result of short-term imbalances of stress and recovery, whereas overtraining is the long-term result. Overtraining causes declines in tissue repair and nervous system function. It can create hormonal imbalances and often results in severe deficiencies of the immune system, leaving the person weaker, chronically fatigued, mentally drained, and prone to illness and injury. Here is where familiarity with the general symptoms of overtraining and those specific to each person you train, as well as your own instinct and common sense, must be applied along with the science of program design. At times, the body simply cannot keep pace with even the best-planned training programs. This is often due to uncontrollable variables in a person's life that gradually or suddenly add more stress to the equation than was anticipated. When life changes such as personal problems, job stress, or illness arise for your client or athlete, more recovery becomes necessary and may require at least a temporary reduction in duration and frequency of routines. Look for decreased performance, lack of motivation, difficulty sleeping, irritability, unexplained weight loss or gain, and frequent injuries as signs that recovery is not sufficient. New routines with less volume or intensity, longer recovery periods between sessions, a temporary break, and a medical exam are proactive ways of addressing overtraining.

As much as possible, plan and adhere to the amount of recovery between sets. The rest periods between sets are as important as the stimulus itself for achieving the neural-metabolic adaptations desired (see table 6.2). As previously stated, more rest is needed when working with higher-intensity sets, which require greater neural drive, than when performing sets with lower intensity, which depend more on metabolic factors for recovery.

If full recovery between sets is not required for goal achievement, then muscles can often recover adequately through active rest, such as by performing supersets or active stretching for muscle groups opposing or unrelated to the ones being targeted. These active rest periods may be a valuable use of training time. They may allow the person to continue to progress toward other training goals or needs, such as increasing mobility, targeting opposing muscle groups, correcting weak links, or simply increasing overall volume for metabolic and hypertrophy purposes.

Sequence

Sequence is the specific planned exercise order in a given routine. It is the program variable that must allow for the largest amount of random change in a training program. This is due to the numerous uncontrollable variables that can influence exercise sequence. For example, having less time than planned for the training session, training at a different facility with different equipment, having broken equipment, dealing with a recent strain or injury, or simply having to work among and share equipment with other people in a crowded gym are just a few of the situations that can force a change of the routine and interrupt the planned exercise sequence.

An exercise is immediately affected once it is moved from its originally designed sequence; in turn, it will affect others. For example, imagine that the barbell squat exercise is planned for the first circuit but is not available until much later in the routine after other leg and back work had been performed. The other leg and back exercises would probably seem easier, and obviously the intensity and perhaps even the volume of the barbell squat would probably need to be decreased. However, changes in volume should be kept within the planned training parameters when possible to allow pursuit of the proper neural-metabolic adaptations desired in the current phase of the program cycle.

Numerous guidelines found in literature and applied in practice may be helpful for designing efficient sequencing of exercise routines (see list below). Remember that these are only guidelines, not rules. Experienced and advanced athletes with higher levels of neuromuscular efficiency can purposely go outside most guidelines to accomplish different training effects. There are valid reasons for ignoring any guideline for the right person and for the proper goal.

1. Place exercises of high neurological challenge and demand (such as those with greater stability and balance demand) before those of low demand.

2. Place high-priority exercises before those of lower priority, such as training general movement pattern exercises before isolated movements.

3. Place new exercises with higher motor learning requirements before ones previously mastered or with low motor learning requirements.

4. Place high-intensity exercises before those of lower intensity, and place those planned for application of heavy loads and multiple sets before supplemental exercises.

5. Place exercises targeting stabilizers (such as rotator cuff, ankle supinators, and specific core work) at the end of the routine.

Periodization and Program Design

The key to designing effective short-, medium-, and long-term resistance exercise programs is to develop a system that efficiently plans, organizes, and manages all exercise variables. Periodization is a system of program design that sets appropriate cycles and phases, organizes routines, and manipulates all acute variables of exercise. Theories and definitions of periodization vary widely, but the basic concepts have been time tested for success and have been used by trainers and strength coaches since the early 1950s. The origin of periodization is credited to professionals in Russia and other Eastern Bloc countries. It was later adopted by those in the United States who had witnessed the superior performances of other countries' athletes in world competition.

Much research has shown the ability of periodization to produce significantly better results than straight-set training or linear progression models. This comes as no surprise because a continual variety of training stimuli are needed in order for the neuromuscular system to continue to progress after initial adaptations have taken place. Planning, organizing, and managing training stimuli and manipulating program variables in a systematic manner are what define periodization. Much of this information has already been provided, leaving only the need to discuss the planning of program cycles and organization of training phases in ways that will make the overall program effective in accomplishing goals and addressing needs.

Program Cycles

A resistance exercise program should be considered as always ongoing but should be broken down into long- and short-term blocks, or periods of time, that are termed cycles. Breaking a program into cycles is helpful for prioritizing training goals and needs. Cycles can vary greatly in the amount of time they span. They are designed to apply more focus on certain goals and needs while placing less attention on others based on established priorities. Macrocycles are long-term cycles that may encompass several months to a year and help to set the priorities and time lines in which to accomplish training goals or address individual needs. Macrocycles will need to be further broken down into more manageable segments called mesocycles. Mesocycles enable a person to track progress, reassess goals and needs, design new routines, and make any needed adjustments in order to stay on the time lines set forth by the macrocycle. Mesocycles can also vary widely in length, usually ranging from 3 to 12 weeks. I have found that 6- to 8-week mesocycles work well for most people. This is enough time for an athlete to experience significant and measurable results yet not become bored or frustrated with the current routines. This time frame is frequent enough to allow you to identify and correct problems that may have recently surfaced before they can inhibit further progress. You should reassess and gather as much pertinent data as possible between mesocycles to help you select exercises and build the routines that will make up the next mesocycle.

Training Phases

Mesocycles focus on certain priorities, but all other goals or needs should not be ignored in the process. Other than competitive athletes who may need to focus on only a specific set of biomotor abilities while ignoring others, most people could benefit from improvements in all base biomotor abilities as well as make progress in reaching aesthetic goals as well. Therefore, the average person who decides to spend a six- to eight-week mesocycle completely focusing on maximal strength gains may also lose endurance or mobility and even muscle size while also gaining body fat unless some degree of attention is also directed to these areas as well. Balancing priorities within a mesocycle is what training phases are designed to do.

Many experts believe that it is ineffective to attempt to improve on every biomotor ability simultaneously during each training routine, because there is not enough time in a 30- to 60-minute session to adequately apply and adapt to that much varied stimuli. Therefore, a mesocycle can be divided into training phases lasting one to three weeks that focus on only certain neural-metabolic adaptations. These shorter time periods allow for progress in one area without any significant loss in others. However, training phases must be planned appropriately throughout the mesocycle to ensure that all priorities are addressed. The following are sample types of training phases that could be strategically placed throughout a mesocycle to address specific priorities.

- *Transitional phase.* This phase is typically the first week of a mesocycle and is characterized by low-intensity and low-volume training. This phase is commonly used in beginning a mesocycle when the previous mesocycle ended with a high-intensity strength or power phase. During this week, athletes undergo assessments to measure progress and to identify any adaptations achieved in the previous mesocycle. The trainer designs a new program with an emphasis on training technique, and the trainer introduces it to the athlete. The athlete learns new movement patterns and practices the planned exercise sequence. The athlete and trainer also review nutritional strategies with their trainer. The recommended volume for this phase is 1 or 2 sets per exercise for about 10 to 12 repetitions.

• *Endurance phase.* This phase typically consists of lower-intensity and higher-volume routines. Muscular and cardiovascular endurance is the primary focus. However, this is also a logical phase for focusing on repetitive performance of new or difficult exercises because the intensity loads are low, which will help the athlete with attempting to master new movement patterns. Exercises that require different stabilization strategies or have high balance demands are ideal for additional practice during these phases. Further descriptive titles can be used for a phase if endurance weeks are combined with other complementary phases, such as a transitional-endurance phase or an endurance-hypertrophy phase. Volume recommendations range from 1 to 3 sets for about 15 to 20 reps per exercise but occasionally are prescribed with as high as 50 reps in extreme cases.

• *Hypertrophy phase.* This phase is designed to apply the greatest combinations of intensity and volume in order to elicit muscle hypertrophy (muscle growth). The overlap of increased intensity and the maintenance of high to moderate volume also makes this phase highly metabolic and induces greater hormonal responses than other training phases, making it great for reduction of body fat as well as hypertrophy. Hypertrophy phases can be appropriate even for those people not interested in large increases of muscle mass, as long as exercise selection and volume for specific muscles are properly planned. Recommendations for sets and repetitions span from 3 to 5 sets per exercise for 8 to 15 repetitions. Hypertrophy training covers a wide range of time under tension, so more descriptive titles can be used to designate the training priorities, such as hypertrophy endurance phase or hypertrophy strength phase.

• *Strength phase.* This phase is characterized by high levels of intensity and reduced volumes of work. Greater rest periods and slower training tempos are also typically implemented to maximize motor unit recruitment. The strength phase focuses on more neural and intramuscular adaptations than hypertrophy and endurance phases. Stability is a prerequisite for maximal strength; therefore, fewer exercises are selected and fewer positioning options and techniques are used that require high balance demands. Various titles may be used for strength phases that overlap with other training phases, such as strength hypertrophy phase and strength power phase. Volume recommendations are from 5 to 8 sets with 3 to 5 repetitions per exercise. With these recommendations, you can see why most people prefer combinations of hypertrophy and strength because this many sets of heavy loads are often too high risk for perceived benefits.

• *Power phase.* To produce power, the speed or rate of force production is as important, if not more so, as the amount of force produced. For this reason, power phases of training are characterized by the use of moderate-intensity and even low-intensity loads with low volumes of sets and repetitions and faster tempos. Power training is difficult with standard resistance exercise movements because a proportional amount of effort that does not promote gains in power must be spent on decelerating the weight loads. Power training will often incorporate more ballistic movements such as cleans, snatches, plyometric exercises, and medicine-ball throws. Power training exacts a high neural demand for the quick productions and reductions of force, plus the increased need for dynamic stability and balance. Therefore, volume recommendations for power typically range from 3 to 5 sets of 5 to 10 reps.

The division of a macrocycle into manageable mesocycles and the division of mesocycles into the various training phases may seem like a difficult process, but it is well worth the effort. You can do this by clearly identifying the general overall goals that a person would like to achieve for an upcoming year, such as endurance, strength, hypertrophy, or weight loss, which sets the priorities for the macrocycle. The next step is to create specific subgoals that you and the athlete set at reasonable time periods throughout the year in order to begin to design the appropriate mesocycles to achieve the subgoals. Each mesocycle has its priorities set according to the macrocycle, so you can then divide them up into weekly training phases proportionately in order to reach subgoals without losing ground in other areas. Figure 6.1 provides an example of an actual macrocycle that was created for a middle-aged healthy executive who takes fitness seriously. This person's general overall goals include improved conditioning, increased muscularity, improved strength and stability, and enhanced performance in a few recreational athletic activities.

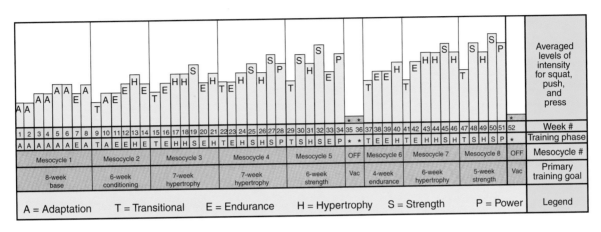

Figure 6.1 Sample macrocycle for balanced fitness.

Sample Routines

It is impossible to design an effective program or even build a simple resistance training routine for any person without first conducting a comprehensive assessment in order to identify the person's training needs. This process may include such features as a total health and medical questionnaire, postural assessment, general movement pattern assessment, gait assessment, cardiorespiratory conditioning tests, and perhaps an isolated joint mobility and stability analysis in order to determine joint integrity and identify specific muscular weaknesses. Without such an assessment, the program would lack information critical for correcting muscular imbalances, regaining posture, improving spinal mechanics, restoring joint function, and gaining awareness of serious health risks.

Therefore, the following sample routines are provided for study purposes and not designed for any specific person. These sample routines will help you see how you can select types and sequences of exercises, build routines, and incorporate and manipulate all other variables throughout a mesocycle. These sample programs are designed in a balanced manner, which typically would not be the case with an actual client. Most people have muscular imbalances, postural deviations, and specific muscular weaknesses that only a well-designed unbalanced program can correct. In more advanced cases, certain manipulations, physical therapy, and tissue work may also be needed for restoring joint function and addressing imbalances. However, for fit and healthy people, these routines, if practiced with the proper technique and within the appropriate intensity and volume, should provide for challenging and safe practical research and help you understand the science and art of program design.

Base Full-Body Routine

Tables 6.3 and 6.4 depict a sample balanced initial full-body routine that addresses frequent needs and common goals of people who have not been training on a regular basis. It is referred to as a base routine because when a person first begins resistance training after a layoff or for the first time, the priority is to establish a fitness base, or foundation, on which all other future routines and programs will be built. Core activation exercises are immediately introduced to help with integration of the suggested breathing methods and to provide for better control of intra-abdominal and intrathoracic pressure for improved trunk stabilization. The trunk, lower-body, and upper-body exercises promote the development of general movement patterns and also target the various subsystems responsible for helping develop better pelvic and spinal stability. Development of good posture and increased spinal control with particular focus on improving lumbar flexion and thoracic extension are also priorities of a base routine. No rotational movements of the spine are yet prescribed because these movements may induce high amounts of compensation in an immobile and unstable spine. The set, repetition, and tempo recommendations are consistent with general strength, conditioning, and stability development, with a chance of providing moderate hypertrophy for those who are at this stage.

Advanced Full-Body Routine

The sample routines in tables 6.5 and 6.6 may be more appropriate for the person who is currently on a regular exercise schedule. For these routines, it is assumed that the person has good development of core control, pelvic and spinal stability, and proficiency in performance of all general movement patterns. Therefore, more attention can be directed to aesthetic-based goals because structural needs have been addressed and a solid fitness base has been established. More challenging compound movements have been added as well as a few isolated movements for certain muscle groups to improve aesthetics and performance. There may need to be a few mesocycles between the base full-body routine and either of these advanced full-body routines. The differences may not be too apparent at first glance, but you will discover them under closer study and quickly realize them if you experiment with them personally.

Advanced Split Routine

If a person is ready to increase training frequency and wants greater amounts of muscle strengthening, hypertrophy, or conditioning, then split routines are the next step. Split routines divide the body into two or more sections to allow more frequent training, increase total volume, and allow for adequate recovery. These routines emphasize training only certain areas of the body while avoiding others. There are many methods of dividing muscle groups into split routines depending on the weekly frequency of training sessions. The example shown in tables 6.7 through 6.10 is a four-day split that uses a push–pull emphasis for designing and splitting the routines. Biceps are switched to push days while triceps are substituted on the pull days in order to provide better arm recovery for pushing and pulling. I call these routines anterior and posterior splits because each routine emphasizes muscle groups on either the front or the back of the body. True push–pull routines and upper–lower routines are also very common examples of four-day-a-week splits that could be tried on different mesocycles. Be sure to follow the listed sequence of each routine even if days are missed, because a person could easily begin training the body in an unbalanced manner if performing more of one split than another.

Tips on Programming and Periodization

When implementing periodization into a client's or athlete's program, remember that you should address the person's health conditions and needs and establish a good base. In the initial phases of training, a person can typically make progress through the use of predetermined and consistent amounts of sets and repetitions while linearly progressing the intensity. This means that the resistance load is increased whenever repetition goals for a given set become easy to accomplish. However, linear progression is most often short lived, and plateaus will eventually occur that will hinder progress or even reverse it.

When you're ready to begin designing periodized workouts, you may wish to start one step at a time for some less experienced people you train. Exercise programming and periodization models are not mastered overnight. Too much variation and random changes can supply an overload of information and apply too much varied stress for the person's neuromuscular system to adapt to, which can be as ineffective as training with no variation at all. Consider these tips on periodization:

1. Break up macrocycles into smaller, more manageable programs or mesocycles.

2. Design each mesocycle with a certain number of the various endurance, hypertrophy, strength, and power phases, depending on specific training goals.

3. Begin each mesocycle with a transitional phase.

4. Practice movements and integrate positioning options that require more stabilization and greater balance demands while intensity is low.

5. Use more stabilized positioning during phases in which increased motor unit recruitment and maximal strength are desired.

6. Keep an inverse relationship between intensity and overall volume.

7. When decreasing repetitions, increase sets, increase rest periods, and select fewer movements for each muscle group.

8. Make small adjustments to the sequence according to the priorities of the training phase.

9. Never compromise structural integrity and overall health needs for the pursuit of specific training goals.

10. Always integrate and adhere to all elements of proper exercise technique. What is done can only be as efficient as how it is done.

Tables 6.3 through 6.10 appear on the following pages.

I hope this book proves to be a valuable resource for you. By learning and following the training principles and exercise techniques presented in this book, you should be able to achieve higher levels of fitness and experience more success in reaching all aesthetic and performance goals for yourself as well as those whom you serve. Remember that you are your first and most important client.

TABLE 6.3 Base Strength Development A

7-week mesocycle PHASE	Week 1 TRANSITIONAL	Week 2 ENDURANCE	Week 3 HYPERTROPHY-ENDURANCE	Week 4 HYPERTROPHY-STRENGTH	Week 5 ENDURANCE	Week 6 HYPERTROPHY	Week 7 HYPERTROPHY-STRENGTH	Notes
Tempo	3121	3121	3121	3121	3121	3121	3121	
Volume: Sets × reps	2 × 10-12	2 × 17-20	1-3 × 12-15	1-4 × 8-10	2 × 17-20	1-3 × 10-12	1-4 × 8-10	
Warm-up	Recumbent bike 10 min Active stretching, Four-Point Core Activation							
FIRST CIRCUIT								
Dumbbell Reverse Lunge	2 × 10-12	2 × 17-20	1 × 12-15	1 × 8-10	2 × 17-20	1 × 10-12	1 × 8-10	Isolateral
Cable One-Arm Decline Horizontal Press	2 × 10-12	2 × 17-20	1 × 12-15	1 × 8-10	2 × 17-20	1 × 10-12	1 × 8-10	Lunge position
Cable Knee Flexion	2 × 10-12	2 × 17-20	1 × 12-15	1 × 8-10	2 × 17-20	1 × 10-12	1 × 8-10	Isolateral
Cable One-Arm Median Row	2 × 10-12	2 × 17-20	1 × 12-15	1 × 8-10	2 × 17-20	1 × 10-12	1 × 8-10	Lunge position
Bench Single Bent-Leg Hip Flexion	2 × 10-12	2 × 17-20	1 × 12-15	1 × 8-10	2 × 17-20	1 × 10-12	1 × 8-10	+ incline = + intensity
SECOND CIRCUIT								
Barbell Squat	2 × 10-12	2 × 17-20	3 × 12-15	3 × 8-10	2 × 17-20	3 × 10-12	3 × 8-10	Shoulder-width stance
Dumbbell Incline Median Press	2 × 10-12	2 × 17-20	3 × 12-15	3 × 8-10	2 × 17-20	3 × 10-12	3 × 8-10	Median plane: see page 208, with bench inclined to 30-45 degrees
Cable One-Arm Frontal Pull-Down	2 × 10-12	2 × 17-20	3 × 12-15	3 × 8-10	2 × 17-20	3 × 10-12	3 × 8-10	Seated
Cable Hip Abduction	2 × 10-12	2 × 17-20	3 × 12-15	3 × 8-10	2 × 17-20	3 × 10-12	3 × 8-10	Alternate each set
Incline Bench Reverse Trunk Flexion	2 × 10-12	2 × 17-20	3 × 12-15	3 × 8-10	2 × 17-20	3 × 10-12	3 × 8-10	+ incline = + intensity
SUPPLEMENTAL								
Cable Shoulder External Rotation	1-2 × 10-12	1-2 × 10-12	1-2 × 10-12	1-2 × 10-12	1-2 × 10-12	1-2 × 10-12	1-2 × 10-12	15 degrees of shoulder abduction

TABLE 6.4　Base Strength Development B

7-week mesocycle	Week 1	Week 2	Week 3	Week 4	Week 5	Week 6	Week 7	Notes
PHASE	TRANSITIONAL	ENDURANCE	HYPERTROPHY-ENDURANCE	HYPERTROPHY-STRENGTH	ENDURANCE	HYPERTROPHY	HYPERTROPHY-STRENGTH	
Tempo	3121	3121	3121	3121	3121	3121	3121	
Volume: Sets × reps	2 × 10-12	2 × 17-20	1-3 × 12-15	1-3 × 8-10	2 × 17-20	1-3 × 10-12	1-4 × 8-10	
Warm-up	Recumbent bike 10 min, Active stretching, Quadraplex							
FIRST CIRCUIT								
Dumbbell Side Lunge	2 × 10-12	2 × 17-20	1 × 12-15	1 × 8-10	2 × 17-20	1 × 10-12	1 × 8-10	Unilateral
Dumbbell One-Arm and One-Leg Frontal Press	2 × 10-12	2 × 17-20	1 × 12-15	1 × 8-10	2 × 17-20	1 × 10-12	1 × 8-10	On one leg, seated when heavy
Cable One-Arm Frontal Pull-Down	2 × 10-12	2 × 17-20	1 × 12-15	1 × 8-10	2 × 17-20	1 × 10-12	1 × 8-10	Lunge position
Cable Knee Extension	2 × 10-12	2 × 17-20	1 × 12-15	1 × 8-10	2 × 17-20	1 × 10-12	1 × 8-10	Unilateral
Cable One-Arm Horizontal Row	2 × 10-12	2 × 17-20	1 × 12-15	1 × 8-10	2 × 17-20	1 × 10-12	1 × 8-10	Lunge position
SECOND CIRCUIT								
Dumbbell Deadlift	2 × 10-12	2 × 17-20	3 × 12-15	3 × 8-10	2 × 17-20	3 × 10-12	4 × 8-10	Wide stance
Dumbbell and Bench Chest Press	2 × 10-12	2 × 17-20	3 × 12-15	3 × 8-10	2 × 17-20	3 × 10-12	4 × 8-10	Try on Swiss ball week 5
Cable Shoulder Extension	2 × 10-12	2 × 17-20	3 × 12-15	3 × 8-10	2 × 17-20	3 × 10-12	4 × 8-10	Standing
Machine Knee Flexion	2 × 10-12	2 × 17-20	3 × 12-15	3 × 8-10	2 × 17-20	3 × 10-12	4 × 8-10	Bilateral
Flat Bench Reverse Trunk Flexion	2 × 10-12	2 × 17-20	3 × 12-15	3 × 8-10	2 × 17-20	3 × 10-12	4 × 8-10	+ incline = + intensity
SUPPLEMENTAL								
Machine Calf Extension	1-2 × 15-17	1-2 × 15-17	1-2 × 15-17	1-2 × 15-17	1-2 × 15-17	1-2 × 15-17	1-2 × 15-17	Substitute 1 set of Machine Tib Flexion
Machine Ankle Flexion	1-2 × 15-17	1-2 × 15-17	1-2 × 15-17	1-2 × 15-17	1-2 × 15-17	1-2 × 15-17	1-2 × 15-17	

TABLE 6.5 *Full-Body Fitness A*

7-week mesocycle	Week 1	Week 2	Week 3	Week 4	Week 5	Week 6	Week 7	Notes
PHASE	TRANSITIONAL	ENDURANCE	HYPERTROPHY-ENDURANCE	HYPERTROPHY-STRENGTH	ENDURANCE	HYPERTROPHY	HYPERTROPHY-STRENGTH	
Tempo	3121	2121	3121	4122	2121	3121	4122	
Volume: Sets × reps	2 × 10-12	2 × 17-20	2-3 × 12-15	1-4 × 8-10	2 × 17-20	2-3 × 10-12	1-4 × 8-10	
Warm-up	Recumbent bike 10 min — Active stretching, Four-Point Core Activation, Quadraplex							
FIRST CIRCUIT								
Dumbbell Side Lunge	2 × 10-12	2 × 17-20	2 × 12-15	1 × 8-10	2 × 17-20	2 × 10-12	1 × 8-10	Isolateral
Cable One-Arm Decline Horizontal Press	2 × 10-12	2 × 17-20	2 × 12-15	1 × 8-10	2 × 17-20	2 × 10-12	1 × 8-10	Lunge position
Cable Knee Flexion	2 × 10-12	2 × 17-20	2 × 12-15	1 × 8-10	2 × 17-20	2 × 10-12	1 × 8-10	Isolateral
Cable One-Arm Median Row	2 × 10-12	2 × 17-20	2 × 12-15	1 × 8-10	2 × 17-20	2 × 10-12	1 × 8-10	Lunge position
Cable Trunk Rotation With Flexion	2 × 10-12	2 × 17-20	2 × 12-15	1 × 8-10	2 × 17-20	2 × 10-12	1 × 8-10	Lunge position
SECOND CIRCUIT								
Barbell Squat	2 × 10-12	2 × 17-20	3 × 12-15	4 × 8-10	2 × 17-20	3 × 10-12	4 × 8-10	Shoulder-width stance
Dumbbell Incline Median Press	2 × 10-12	2 × 17-20	3 × 12-15	4 × 8-10	2 × 17-20	3 × 10-12	4 × 8-10	Median plane; see page 208, with bench inclined to 30-45 degrees
Machine Seated Leg Press	2 × 10-12	2 × 17-20	3 × 12-15	4 × 8-10	2 × 17-20	3 × 10-12	4 × 8-10	Superset wide-narrow
Machine Frontal Pull-Up	2 × 10-12	2 × 17-20	3 × 12-15	4 × 8-10	2 × 17-20	3 × 10-12	4 × 8-10	Emphasis on scapular movement
Cable One-Arm 90-Degree Elbow Extension	2 × 10-12	2 × 17-20	3 × 12-15	4 × 8-10	2 × 17-20	3 × 10-12	4 × 8-10	Lunge position, bilateral
Machine Calf Extension/Tib Flexion	2 × 10-12	2 × 17-20	3 × 12-15	4 × 8-10	2 × 17-20	3 × 10-12	4 × 8-10	Substitute 1 set Machine Ankle Flexion
SUPPLEMENTAL								
Cable Shoulder External Rotation	1-2 × 10-12	1-2 × 10-12	1-2 × 10-12	1-2 × 10-12	1-2 × 10-12	1-2 × 10-12	1-2 × 10-12	15 degrees of shoulder abduction

TABLE 6.6 Full-Body Fitness B

7-week mesocycle PHASE	Week 1 TRANSITIONAL	Week 2 ENDURANCE	Week 3 HYPERTROPHY-ENDURANCE	Week 4 HYPERTROPHY-STRENGTH	Week 5 ENDURANCE	Week 6 HYPERTROPHY	Week 7 HYPERTROPHY-STRENGTH	Notes
Tempo	3121	2121	3121	4122	2121	3121	4122	
Volume: Sets × reps	2 × 10-12	2 × 17-20	2-3 × 12-15	1-4 × 8-10	2 × 17-20	2-3 × 10-12	1-4 × 8-10	
Warm-up				Recumbent bike 10 min / Active stretching, Four-Point Core Activation, Quadraplex				
FIRST CIRCUIT								
Med Ball Traveling Lunge	2 × 10-12	2 × 17-20	2 × 12-15	1 × 8-10	2 × 17-20	2 × 10-12	1 × 8-10	Alternate legs
Dumbbell Swiss Ball One-Arm Horizontal Press	2 × 10-12	2 × 17-20	2 × 12-15	1 × 8-10	2 × 17-20	2 × 10-12	1 × 8-10	Stabilize trunk and neck
Dumbbell Deadlift	2 × 10-12	2 × 17-20	2 × 12-15	1 × 8-10	2 × 17-20	2 × 10-12	1 × 8-10	Wide stance
Cable One-Arm Frontal Pull-Down	2 × 10-12	2 × 17-20	2 × 12-15	1 × 8-10	2 × 17-20	2 × 10-12	1 × 8-10	Lunge position
Cable Hip Abduction	2 × 10-12	2 × 17-20	2 × 12-15	1 × 8-10	2 × 17-20	2 × 10-12	1 × 8-10	Focus on pelvic stabilization
SECOND CIRCUIT								
Dumbbell Reverse Lunge	2 × 10-12	2 × 17-20	3 × 12-15	4 × 8-10	2 × 17-20	3 × 10-12	4 × 8-10	Alternate
Barbell Horizontal Press	2 × 10-12	2 × 17-20	3 × 12-15	4 × 8-10	2 × 17-20	3 × 10-12	4 × 8-10	Keep proper range of motion
Machine Knee Flexion	2 × 10-12	2 × 17-20	3 × 12-15	4 × 8-10	2 × 17-20	3 × 10-12	4 × 8-10	Bilateral
Cable Low Median Row	2 × 10-12	2 × 17-20	3 × 12-15	4 × 8-10	2 × 17-20	3 × 10-12	4 × 8-10	Focus on posture
Machine Ankle Extension	2 × 10-12	2 × 17-20	3 × 12-15	4 × 8-10	2 × 17-20	3 × 10-12	4 × 8-10	Keep reps at the higher range
Dumbbell Median Row	2 × 10-12	2 × 17-20	3 × 12-15	4 × 8-10	2 × 17-20	3 × 10-12	4 × 8-10	Switch to high cable when heavy
Swiss Ball Reverse Trunk Flexion	2 × 10-12	2 × 17-20	3 × 12-15	4 × 8-10	2 × 17-20	3 × 10-12	4 × 8-10	Focus on lumbar flexion

TABLE 6.7 **Anterior Split A**

7-week mesocycle	Week 1	Week 2	Week 3	Week 4	Week 5	Week 6	Week 7	Notes
PHASE	TRANSITIONAL	ENDURANCE	HYPERTROPHY-ENDURANCE	HYPERTROPHY-STRENGTH	ENDURANCE	HYPERTROPHY	STRENGTH	
Tempo	3121	2121	3121	4122	2121	3121	4122	
Volume: Sets × reps	2 × 10-12	2 × 17-20	2-3 × 12-15	1-4 × 8-10	2 × 17-20	2-3 × 10-12	1-4 × 6-10	
Warm-up	Recumbent bike 10 min / Active stretching, Quadraplex, Bent-Leg Raises							
FIRST CIRCUIT								
Dumbbell Side Lunge	2 × 10-12	2 × 17-20	2 × 12-15	2 × 8-10	2 × 17-20	2 × 10-12	2 × 8-10	Isolateral
Cable One-Arm Decline Horizontal Press	2 × 10-12	2 × 17-20	2 × 12-15	2 × 8-10	2 × 17-20	2 × 10-12	2 × 8-10	Lunge position
Cable Knee Extension	2 × 10-12	2 × 17-20	2 × 12-15	2 × 8-10	2 × 17-20	2 × 10-12	2 × 8-10	Flex hip each rep
Cable One-Arm 90-Degree Elbow Flexion	2 × 10-12	2 × 17-20	2 × 12-15	2 × 8-10	2 × 17-20	2 × 10-12	2 × 8-10	Lunge position, isolateral
Cable Trunk Rotation With Flexion	2 × 10-12	2 × 17-20	2 × 12-15	2 × 8-10	2 × 17-20	2 × 10-12	2 × 8-10	Lunge position
SECOND CIRCUIT								
Med Ball Traveling Lunge	2 × 10-12	2 × 17-20	3 × 12-15	Skip	2 × 17-20	3 × 10-12	Skip	Alternate steps
Dumbbell Horizontal Press	2 × 10-12	2 × 17-20	3 × 12-15	4 × 8-10	2 × 17-20	3 × 10-12	4 × 6-8	45-degree, horizontal plane; see page 198 for technique (but adjust bench to 30 to 45 degrees)
Machine Seated Leg Press (high reps)	2 × 15	1 × 35, 1 × 25	1 × 25, 2 × 20	1 × 20, 3 × 15	1 × 35, 1 × 25	1 × 25, 2 × 20	1 × 20, 3 × 15	Follow rep scheme
Dumbbell Incline Median Press	2 × 10-12	2 × 17-20	3 × 12-15	4 × 8-10	2 × 17-20	3 × 10-12	4 × 6-8	Median plane
Dumbbell 15-Degree Elbow Flexion With Supination	2 × 10-12	2 × 17-20	3 × 12-15	4 × 8-10	2 × 17-20	3 × 10-12	4 × 6-8	With supination
Swiss Ball Reverse Trunk Flexion	2 × 10-12	2 × 17-20	3 × 12-15	4 × 8-10	2 × 17-20	3 × 10-12	4 × 6-8	Focus on lumbar flexion
SUPPLEMENTAL								
Machine Ankle Flexion	1-2 × 12-15	1-2 × 12-15	1-2 × 12-15	1-2 × 12-15	1-2 × 12-15	1-2 × 12-15	1-2 × 12-15	

TABLE 6.8 **Posterior Split A**

7-week mesocycle	Week 1	Week 2	Week 3	Week 4	Week 5	Week 6	Week 7	Notes
PHASE	TRANSITIONAL	ENDURANCE	HYPERTROPHY-ENDURANCE	HYPERTROPHY-STRENGTH	ENDURANCE	HYPERTROPHY	STRENGTH	
Tempo	3121	2121	3121	4122	2121	3121	4122	
Volume: Sets × reps	2 × 10-12	2 × 17-20	2-3 × 12-15	1-4 × 8-10	2 × 17-20	2-3 × 10-12	1-4 × 8-10	
Warm-up	Recumbent bike 10 min — Active stretching, Four-Point Core Activation, Quadraplex							
FIRST CIRCUIT								
Cable Knee Flexion	2 × 10-12	2 × 17-20	2 × 12-15	2 × 8-10	2 × 17-20	2 × 10-12	2 × 8-10	Extend hip each rep
Cable One-Arm Median Row	2 × 10-12	2 × 17-20	2 × 12-15	2 × 8-10	2 × 17-20	2 × 10-12	2 × 8-10	Lunge position
Cable Hip Abduction	2 × 10-12	2 × 17-20	2 × 12-15	2 × 8-10	2 × 17-20	2 × 10-12	2 × 8-10	Pelvic stabilization
Cable One-Arm Horizontal Row	2 × 10-12	2 × 17-20	2 × 12-15	2 × 8-10	2 × 17-20	2 × 10-12	2 × 8-10	Lunge position
Cable One-Arm 90-Degree Elbow Extension	2 × 10-12	2 × 17-20	2 × 12-15	2 × 8-10	2 × 17-20	2 × 10-12	2 × 8-10	Lunge position
SECOND CIRCUIT								
45-Degree Hip Extension	2 × 10-12	2 × 17-20	3 × 12-15	4 × 8-10	2 × 17-20	3 × 10-12	4 × 8-10	Alternate
Machine Frontal Pull-Up	2 × 10-12	2 × 17-20	3 × 12-15	4 × 8-10	2 × 17-20	3 × 10-12	4 × 8-10	Emphasis on scapular movement
Machine Knee Flexion	2 × 10-12	2 × 17-20	3 × 12-15	4 × 8-10	2 × 17-20	3 × 10-12	4 × 8-10	Bilateral
Dumbbell Median Row	2 × 10-12	2 × 17-20	3 × 12-15	4 × 8-10	2 × 17-20	3 × 10-12	4 × 8-10	Switch to high cable when heavy
Cable Zero-Degree Elbow Extension	2 × 10-12	2 × 17-20	3 × 12-15	4 × 8-10	2 × 17-20	3 × 10-12	4 × 8-10	Emphasis on scapular positioning
Machine Ankle Extension	2 × 10-12	2 × 17-20	3 × 12-15	4 × 8-10	2 × 17-20	3 × 10-12	4 × 8-10	Keep reps at the higher range
SUPPLEMENTAL								
Cable Shoulder External Rotation	1-2 × 10-12	1-2 × 10-12	1-2 × 10-12	1-2 × 10-12	1-2 × 10-12	1-2 × 10-12	1-2 × 10-12	15 degrees of shoulder abduction

TABLE 6.9 Anterior Split B

7-week mesocycle	Week 1	Week 2	Week 3	Week 4	Week 5	Week 6	Week 7	Notes
PHASE	TRANSITIONAL	ENDURANCE	HYPERTROPHY-ENDURANCE	HYPERTROPHY-STRENGTH	ENDURANCE	HYPERTROPHY	STRENGTH	
Tempo	3121	2121	3121	4122	2121	3121	4122	
Volume: Sets × reps	2 × 10-12	2 × 17-20	2-3 × 12-15	1-4 × 8-10	2 × 17-20	2-3 × 10-12	1-4 × 6-10	
Warm-up	Recumbent bike 10 min Active stretching, Quadraplex, Bent-Leg Raises							
FIRST CIRCUIT								
Dumbbell Reverse Lunge	2 × 10-12	2 × 17-20	2 × 12-15	2 × 8-10	2 × 17-20	2 × 10-12	2 × 8-10	Bilateral
Dumbbell One-Arm and One-Leg Frontal Press	2 × 10-12	2 × 17-20	2 × 12-15	2 × 8-10	2 × 17-20	2 × 10-12	2 × 8-10	Seated, frontal plane
Barbell Hang Clean	2 × 10-12	2 × 10-12	2 × 10-12	2 × 10-12	2 × 10-12	2 × 10-12	2 × 10-12	Focus on technique
Swiss Ball Double-Leg Hip Flexion	2 × 10-12	2 × 17-20	2 × 12-15	2 × 8-10	2 × 17-20	2 × 10-12	2 × 8-10	Single or double
Swiss Ball Trunk Flexion	2 × 10-12	2 × 17-20	2 × 12-15	2 × 8-10	2 × 17-20	2 × 10-12	2 × 8-10	
SECOND CIRCUIT								
Barbell Squat (high reps)	2 × 20	1 × 35, 1 × 25	1 × 25, 2 × 20	1 × 20, 3 × 15	1 × 35, 1 × 25	1 × 20, 2 × 15	1 × 15, 3 × 10	
Incline Bench Reverse Trunk Flexion	2 × 10-12	2 × 17-20	3 × 12-15	4 × 8-10	2 × 17-20	3 × 10-12	4 × 6-8	
Dumbbell and Bench Chest Press	2 × 10-12	2 × 17-20	3 × 12-15	4 × 8-10	2 × 17-20	3 × 10-12	4 × 6-8	
Machine Knee Extension	2 × 12-15	2 × 12-15	2 × 12-15	Skip	2 × 12-15	2 × 12-15	Skip	
Machine Trunk Rotation	2 × 10-12	2 × 17-20	3 × 12-15	4 × 8-10	2 × 17-20	3 × 10-12	4 × 6-8	
Dumbbell 15-Degree Elbow Flexion With Supination	2 × 10-12	2 × 17-20	3 × 12-15	4 × 8-10	2 × 17-20	3 × 10-12	4 × 6-8	Alternate movement
SUPPLEMENTAL								
Squat Rack Push-Up	1-2 sets to failure	1-2 sets to failure	1-2 sets to failure	1-2 sets to failure	1-2 sets to failure	1-2 sets to failure	1-2 sets to failure	

PART III

Exercises

Part III provides a sampling of resistance training exercises that can be used for training any and all areas of the body in a safe manner. These exercises provide clear examples of movements that target either specific muscle groups or larger muscular subsystems. Some exercises are isolated, and specific movement patterns can be used to address a specific performance need or accomplish an aesthetic goal. Other exercises are compound movements that use and develop general movement patterns, many of which can be used to improve the function of the body as it is designed to move in the natural environment and in all three planes.

The names of exercises in this book are unique and were developed through the application of common joint motion terminology. For isolated joint motion exercises, each exercise name begins with the modality (such as a dumbbell, barbell, cable, machine, or Swiss ball). Second, the targeted joint is identified. Third, the actual resisted joint motion is named. For example, what may be referred to as *dumbbell biceps curl* and a *quadriceps extension* is listed as a *dumbbell elbow flexion* and *machine knee extension* in this text. This is preferred when teaching fitness professionals because using a muscle group as part of the name of an exercise often wrongly implies that it may be the only muscle group at work. The fact is there are always numerous muscles working synergistically to produce any motion. Also, if a joint can move in more than one plane, the dominant plane of motion is included in the exercise name. For example, what might be called a *dumbbell pec fly* in one book is known as a *dumbbell shoulder horizontal adduction* herein. This extra descriptive word within the name of the exercise will help you to link kinetic terminology such as *flexion, extension, adduction, abduction,* and *rotation* with their various planes of movement.

For compound movements, we use a similar system for creating logical exercise names. The first word describes the modality of resistance; the second word gives the dominant plane of movement; and the third word describes the general movement, such as *squat, lunge, press, pull,* or *row.* For example, a common exercise that uses a barbell and is aimed at developing the chest musculature is often simply called a *bench press* (which is a strange name since the bench is not what is being "pressed"). This same exercise is called the *barbell, horizontal press* in this book. Other descriptive words that denote a modification, such as *low, high, incline, decline, side, anterior,* and *posterior,* can be interjected to provide a more accurate picture of how the exercise is designed to be performed. Though not perfect, this system of naming exercises integrates an educational approach and provides for a consistent and replicable method that can easily be learned and passed on by fitness professionals in order to better communicate with one another and with clients.

CHAPTER 7

Core and Trunk Exercises

This chapter presents several exercises that target and strengthen the core and trunk muscles. Core control and activation, along with the integration of the suggested breathing method, are particularly important elements of technique for these exercises. The exercise selections can be classified in two general categories—those that develop the ability to stabilize the spine and pelvis, and those that develop the ability to move the spine. Spinal structure and function, as well as specific muscle physiology and all biomechanical factors, were considered when developing the instructions for all elements of technique such as alignment, positioning, motion, stabilization, and suggested breathing method.

These exercise selections vary in their difficulty of stabilization or movement demands in order to provide a well-balanced collection of movements to challenge individuals of all strength and fitness levels. Some exercises are more suited for addressing performance-based goals while others are ideal for achieving more aesthetic-based goals. Variations and modifications that will increase or decrease the level of challenge are also provided in the description section for many exercises. Consider the steps below when selecting exercises as they were derived through combining information relative to exercise technique presented in chapter 4 along with the exercise selection process presented in chapter 5 in order to help select and instruct the efficient performance of each exercise.

1. Identify the goal (aesthetic- or performance-based)
2. Select the desired movement pattern (general movement pattern or specific movement pattern)
3. Select the muscle groups to be targeted (muscle synergies or isolated muscles)
4. Identify alignment of the forces (pull of the muscles vs. pull or push of the resistance)
5. Consider the positioning options (proprioception vs. neural availability)
6. Focus on stabilization (more important than the actual movement)
7. Use and control the planned tempo (affects type of strength, is a component of volume)
8. Integrate breathing method or control

Four-Point Core Activation

The Four-Point Core Activation is a beginning spinal stabilization exercise. This exercise is designed to provide the most neurologically advantageous position to learn core activation and develop strength and control of the transverse abdominis. The direct gravitational pull on the viscera provides for the best proprioception for activation of the core muscles and provides an internal resistance for the transverse abdominis to work against. This exercise can be progressed by elevating an arm or leg to move to a three-point position; it can then be further progressed by adding actual movement of the limb, while coordinating tempo with the breathing method.

Target Muscles

Core (transverse abdominis, diaphragm, pelvic floor muscles, and transversospinalis group)

Joint Motions

None

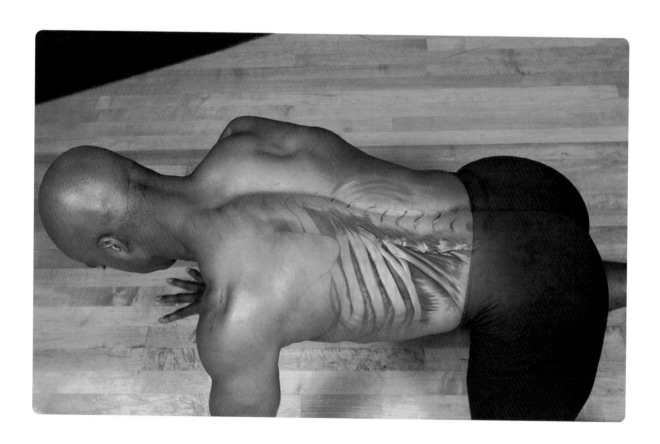

Alignment and Positioning

1. Assume a position on the hands and knees, with the knees placed directly below the hips, the hands directly below the shoulders, and the elbows slightly bent.

2. Position the spine in optimal posture, and hold the head in a neutral position with the eyes looking straight down.

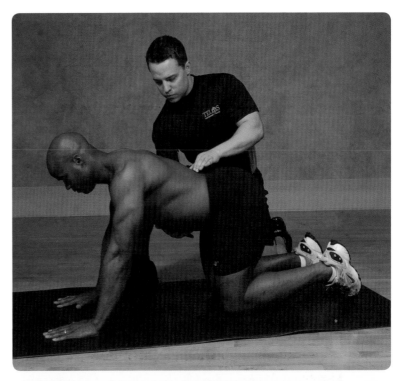

Motion and Stabilization

1. Begin to inhale and allow the abdominal area to distend without losing the posture position of the spine.

2. Slowly breathe out and contract the transverse abdominis by pulling the belly button up toward the spine. Focus on stabilizing the spine and pelvis.

3. Exhale all remaining air while continuing to tighten the abdominal wall and stabilize the spine. Slowly begin to inhale and repeat.

Trainer Techniques

1. Monitor spine and pelvic positioning

2. Cue transverse abdominis (TVA) and cocontractions of the multifidus

3. Spot under the rib cage

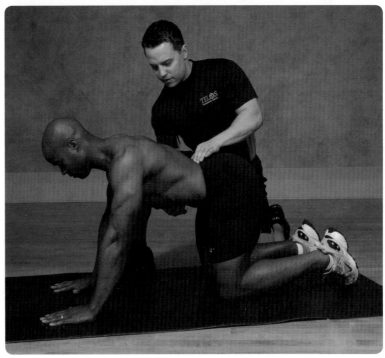

Quadraplex

The Quadraplex can also be considered a "two-point core activation" exercise with added movement of the arm and contralateral leg. The required muscle actions of the shoulder and hip to move and decelerate the limbs, along with the increased demand on the trunk and core muscles for stabilization, make this exercise an advanced progression in core training. Keep in mind that the focus should be placed on stabilization of the spine and pelvis and on the core activation as opposed to the limb movements. To decrease the challenge of the exercise, simply have the athlete hold the arm and leg in the up position rather than raising and lowering them.

Target Muscles

Core (transverse abdominis, diaphragm, pelvic floor muscles, and transversospinalis group), contralateral hip extensors and shoulder flexors, contralateral hip abductors and scapular stabilizers

Joint Motions

Shoulder flexion and hip extension

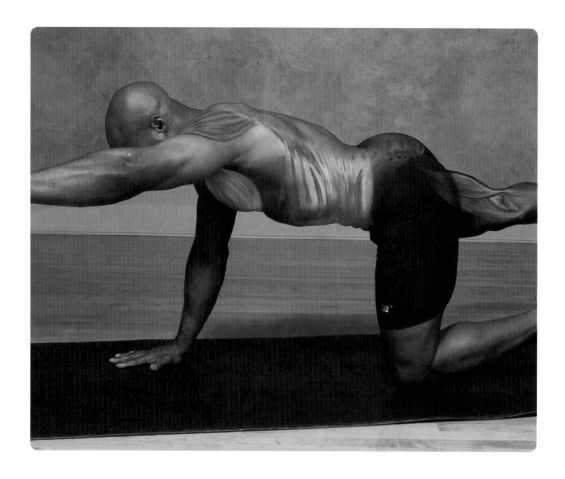

Alignment and Positioning

1. Start on the hands and knees with one knee placed directly below the hip and the opposite hand directly below the shoulder. Place the opposite leg and arm straight out from the body and just off the ground.

2. Slowly draw a deep breath and allow the abdominal area to distend while maintaining posture in the spine and keeping the head in a neutral position.

Motion and Stabilization

1. Slowly begin to exhale, and draw the belly button to the spine while raising the arm and opposite leg without losing optimal posture of the spine or positioning of the pelvis.

2. Hold the top position while continuing to contract the transverse abdominis and stabilizing the spine in optimal posture.

3. Slowly begin to inhale, allowing the abdominal area to distend and the leg and arm to lower while maintaining posture.

Trainer Techniques

1. Monitor spine and pelvic positioning

2. Cue TVA and cocontractions of the multifidus

3. Spot under the rib cage and under the leg

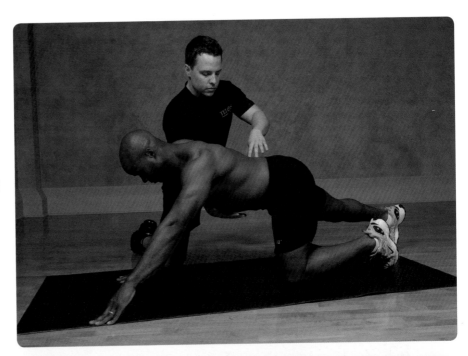

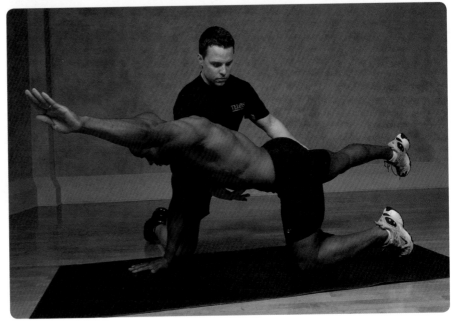

Bent-Leg Raises

This exercise trains core activation in a supine position. The added action of the hip flexor muscles, combined with the inertia of the moving leg, make this exercise substantially more demanding on the core and trunk muscles for stabilization of the spine while still encouraging proper respiratory functions. As with any supine exercise, the upward distension of the viscera is directly resisted by gravity, presenting a greater challenge for diaphragmatic action. This exercise can be progressed by increasing the incline position of the body, straightening the leg, or using faster tempos and leg movement. This exercise may also be performed on a Swiss ball for an increased stabilization challenge.

Target Muscles

Core (transverse abdominis, diaphragm, pelvic floor muscles, and transversospinalis group), spinal flexors, hip flexors

Joint Motions

Hip flexion

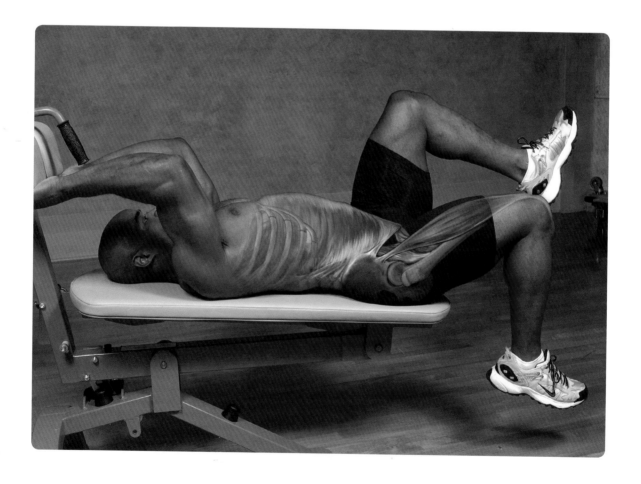

Alignment and Positioning

1. Lie supine while in good posture, with a natural arch in the lower spine and the knees bent and held directly above the hips.

Motion and Stabilization

1. Draw a deep breath, causing the abdominal area to slightly distend upward, with the spine held firm in posture. Slowly lower one leg, keeping the knee in a bent position.

2. Hold, then slowly begin to exhale and draw the belly button toward the spine while raising the leg back up to the starting position and maintaining the natural arch in the lower spine.

Trainer Techniques

1. Monitor spine and pelvic positioning, leg movement

2. Cue TVA, abdominals, and hip flexors

3. Spot under the leg

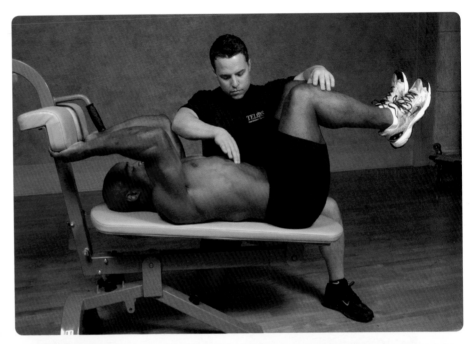

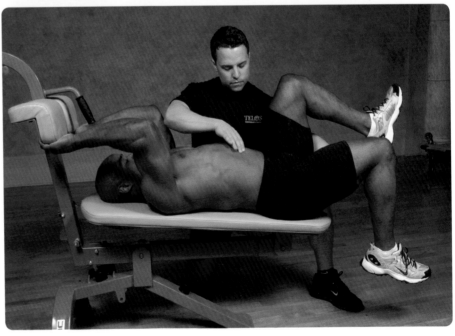

Incline Bench Trunk Flexion

This exercise targets the abdominal and oblique musculature and trains flexion of the spine in a gravity-assisted position. The incline angle and stable bench allow the lifter to more easily achieve his or her maximal amount of spinal flexion. Variations in the amount of incline can be used to increase or decrease resistance as desired. Depending on the lifter's ability and goals, altering leg position to increase or decrease hip flexor involvement is also a viable option.

Target Muscles

Spinal flexors (rectus abdominis, obliques)

Joint Motions

Trunk flexion

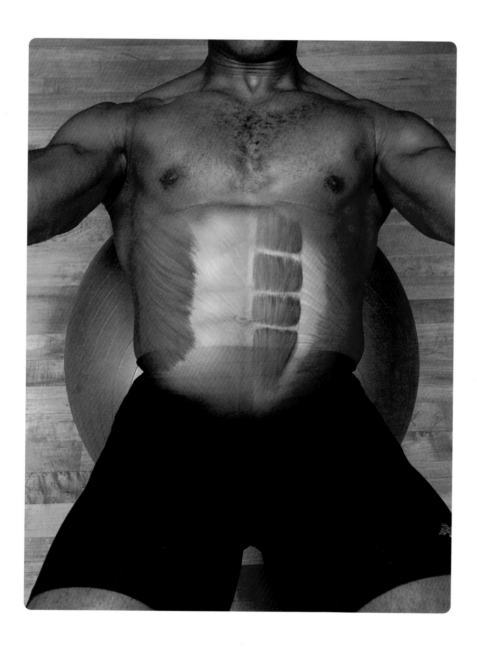

Incline Bench Trunk Flexion

Alignment and Positioning

1. Lie supine on the inclined bench, with the feet braced lightly on the anchor pad or wall, and with the hips and knees bent about 60 and 90 degrees, respectively.

2. Spread the legs so the feet are angled out about 45 degrees (or at about 2 and 10 o'clock).

3. Place the fists under the chin and begin with a full breath of air, the shoulders just off the bench, and tension on the abdominal muscles.

Motion and Stabilization

1. Slowly begin to exhale and pull the ribs toward the pelvis, attempting to move one vertebra at a time.

2. Hold the top position while continuing to exhale, contracting the abdominal muscles, and stabilizing the neck.

3. Slowly begin to inhale, and lower the torso back down to the starting position while stabilizing the head position and maintaining tension on the abdominal muscles.

Trainer Techniques

1. Monitor spine and head positioning, thoracic movement

2. Cue abdominals, obliques

3. Spot under mid back or help support head

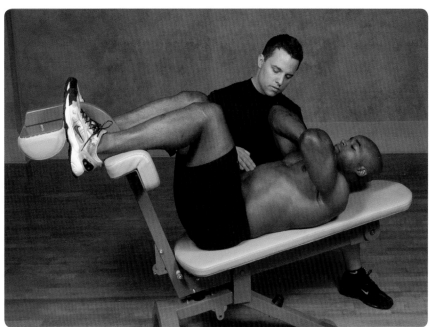

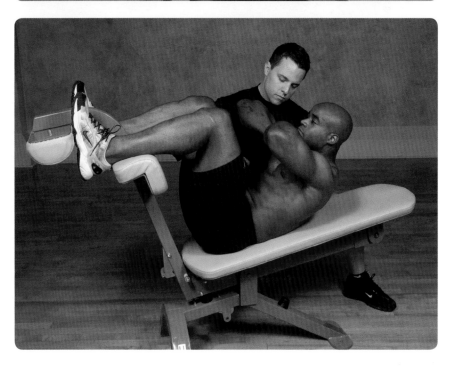

Swiss Ball Trunk Flexion

The shape and yielding surface of the Swiss ball allow for a greater degree of motion because the spine can begin in a position of extension. This exercise targets the abdominal and oblique musculature to flex the spine; it requires greater core and trunk muscle demand as compared to performing this movement on a bench and therefore presents moderate balance challenges. Different angles of resistance can be applied by simply repositioning the body on the ball. Shifting the body down on the ball creates more of an incline angle and decreases resistance. Shifting more of the lower back and pelvis onto the ball flattens out the angle of pull and increases the resistance.

Target Muscles

Spinal flexors (rectus abdominis, obliques)

Joint Motions

Trunk flexion

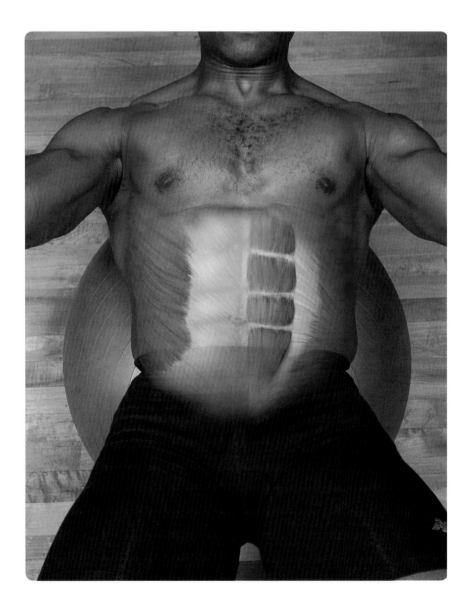

Alignment and Positioning

1. Lie supine on the ball with the feet spread and placed on the floor.

2. Adjust the desired angle on the ball, and let the spine bend back over the ball as available and comfortable for the spine.

3. Place the fists just under the chin, and begin with a full breath of air and with tension on the abdominal muscles.

Motion and Stabilization

1. Slowly begin to exhale, and pull the ribs toward the pelvis, attempting to move one vertebra at a time.

2. Hold the top position while continuing to exhale, contracting the abdominal muscles, and relaxing the neck.

3. Slowly begin to inhale, and lower the torso back down to the starting position while maintaining the head position and keeping tension on the abdominal muscles.

Trainer Techniques

1. Monitor spine and head positioning, thoracic movement

2. Cue abdominals, obliques

3. Spot under mid back or help support head

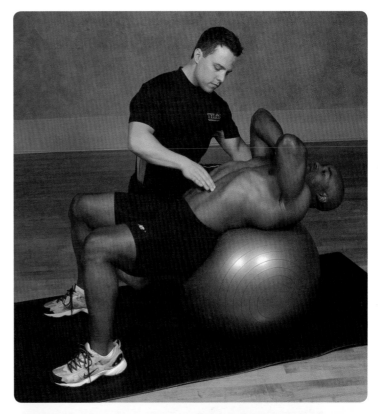

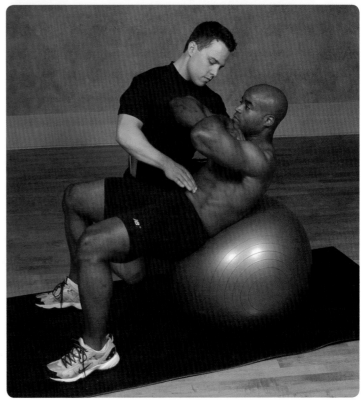

Incline Bench Reverse Trunk Flexion

This exercise targets the abdominal and oblique musculature and trains flexion of the spine in a reverse movement. The reverse trunk flexion contracts the abdominal muscles in an insertion-to-origin pattern opposite that of trunk flexion exercises. This movement also targets flexion of the lumbar region of the spine rather than the flexion of the thoracic region produced from a typical trunk flexion exercise. Different angles of incline or decline can be used with an adjustable bench to increase or decrease resistance.

Target Muscles

Spinal flexors (rectus abdominis, obliques)

Joint Motions

Trunk flexion (lumbar region)

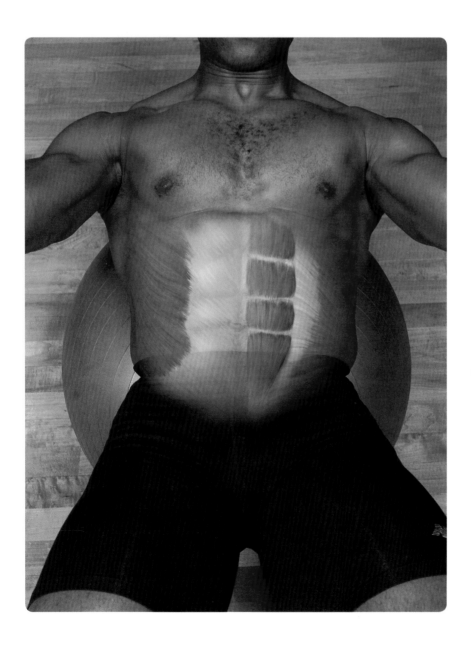

Incline Bench Reverse Trunk Flexion

Alignment and Positioning

1. Lie supine on the bench with the hips and knees bent about 90 degrees.

2. Anchor the body with the arms, and begin with the head just off the pad to target the neck flexors as well as the trunk flexors.

3. Posteriorly tilt the pelvis to flatten the lower back. Begin with a full breath of air and with tension on the abdominal muscles.

Motion and Stabilization

1. Slowly begin to exhale and pull the pelvis toward the ribs, attempting to move one vertebra at a time.

2. Hold the top position while continuing to exhale, contracting the abdominal muscles, and stabilizing the head in a slightly flexed position.

3. Slowly begin to inhale while lowering the pelvis back down to the starting position and maintaining tension on the abdominal muscles. Note: The head can rest on the bench if the neck flexors become fatigued.

Trainer Techniques

1. Monitor spine and pelvic positioning, lumbar movement

2. Cue abdominals, obliques

3. Spot under sacrum

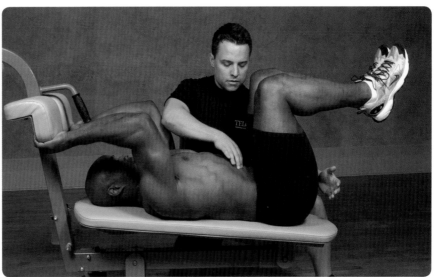

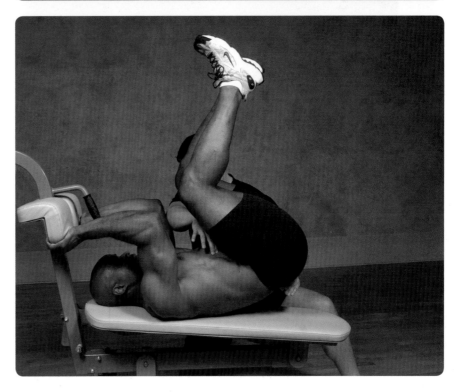

Swiss Ball Reverse Trunk Flexion

This exercise targets the abdominal and oblique musculature and trains flexion of the spine in a reverse movement. Contracting the abdominal muscles in an insertion-to-origin pattern may develop an initial, and possibly increased, activation of the lower fibers of the rectus abdominis. Use of the ball requires additional core and trunk muscle recruitment to correct for balance challenges, and it increases the range of motion by allowing the spine to begin in a position of extension. Increased resistance can be applied by simply repositioning the body on the ball. Shifting the body down on the ball creates more of an incline angle and increases resistance, while shifting more of the lower back and pelvis onto the ball decreases resistance.

Target Muscles

Spinal flexors (rectus abdominis, obliques)

Joint Motions

Trunk flexion (lumbar region)

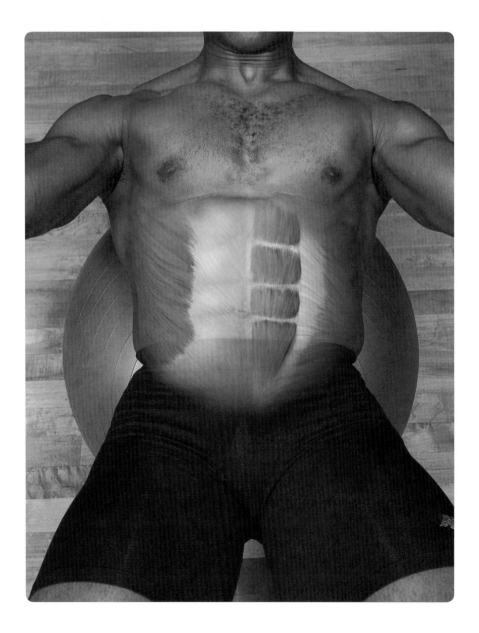

Alignment and Positioning

1. Lie supine on the ball with the hips and knees bent about 90 degrees.

2. Anchor the body with the arms, and begin with the spine pressed against and extended over the ball as available and comfortable for the spine.

3. Begin with a full breath of air, the head held in a neutral position, and tension on the abdominal muscles.

Motion and Stabilization

1. Slowly begin to exhale and pull the pelvis toward the ribs, attempting to move one vertebra at a time.

2. Hold the top position while continuing to exhale, contracting the abdominal muscles, and stabilizing the head in a slightly flexed position.

3. Slowly begin to inhale, and lower the pelvis back down to the starting position while maintaining tension on the abdominal muscles.

Trainer Techniques

1. Monitor spine and pelvic positioning, lumbar movement

2. Cue abdominals, obliques

3. Spot under sacrum

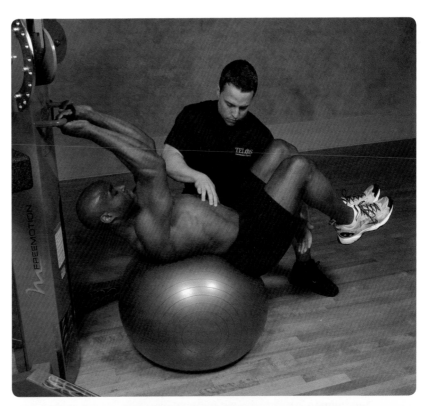

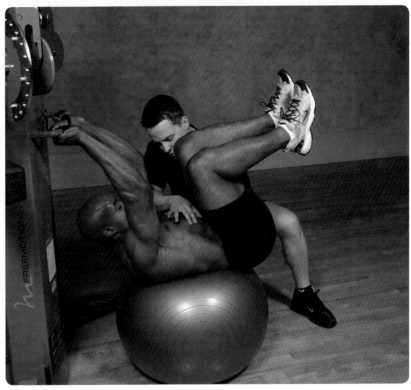

Incline Bench Trunk Extension

This exercise targets the spinal extensors, particularly those of the thoracic region, with some hip extensor assistance. Using a stable bench allows the lifter to more specifically control the degree and region of spinal movement. It is often difficult for some individuals to produce extension of the mid and upper back without hyperextending the lower back. Variations in the amount of incline can be used to increase or decrease resistance as desired. Altering leg position to increase or decrease hip extensor involvement is also a viable option.

Target Muscles

Spinal erectors (iliocostalis, longissimus, spinalis), transversospinalis group

Joint Motions

Trunk extension (thoracic region)

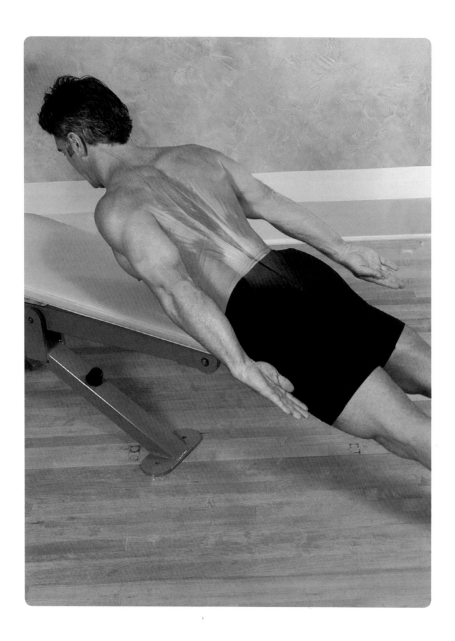

Incline Bench Trunk Extension

Alignment and Positioning

1. Lie prone on the inclined bench with the legs spread comfortably and the feet braced against the floor.

2. Place the arms against the body, out to the sides, or overhead depending on the desired resistance and your level of strength. Begin with a full breath of air, the chest just off the bench, and with tension on the extensors.

Motion and Stabilization

1. Slowly begin to exhale. Activate the core to pull the abdomen slightly off the bench while pulling the shoulder blades back and together.

2. Continue to exhale and attempt to extend the thoracic spine one vertebra at a time without hyperextending the lower back. Then hold the top position and further contract the core.

3. Slowly begin to inhale, and lower the torso back down to the starting position while maintaining the head position and keeping tension on the extensors.

Trainer Techniques

1. Monitor spine and pelvic positioning, thoracic and scapular movement

2. Cue spinal erectors

3. Spot under rib cage

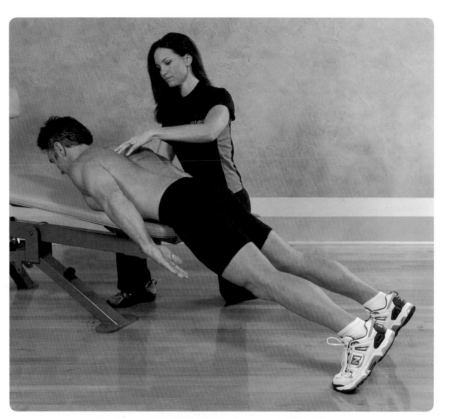

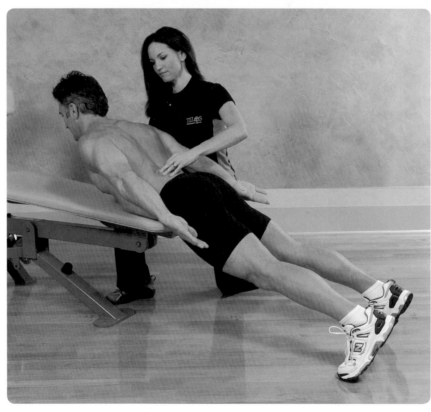

Swiss Ball Trunk Extension

This exercise targets the spinal extensors, particularly those in the thoracic region, with some hip extensor assistance. Using a ball and beginning in a position of spinal flexion can increase the range of motion. The ball also requires some different core, trunk, and hip musculature recruitment to correct for tilting-response challenges. Variations in the angle and weight load can be made by adjusting the body position on the ball. Depending on the lifter's ability and goals, altering leg positions to increase or decrease hip extensor involvement is also a viable option.

Target Muscles

Spinal erectors (iliocostalis, longissimus, spinalis), transversospinalis group

Joint Motions

Trunk extension (thoracic region)

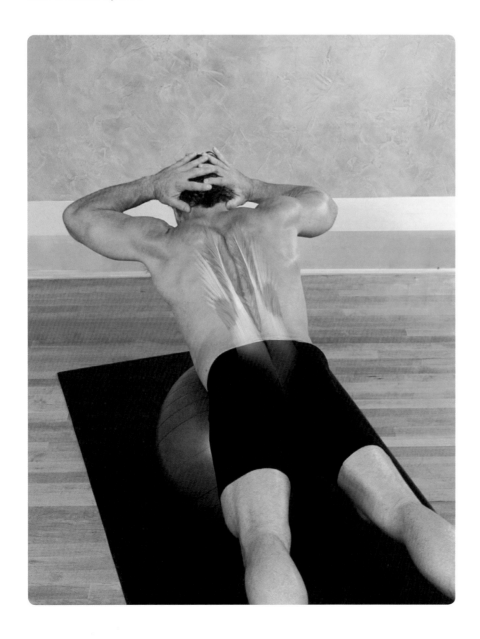

Alignment and Positioning

1. Lie prone on the ball with the legs spread comfortably and the feet braced against the floor.

2. Bend the spine comfortably over the ball, and place the arms against the body, out to the sides, or overhead depending on the desired resistance.

3. Begin with a full breath of air, the chest just off the ball, and with tension on the extensors.

Motion and Stabilization

1. Slowly begin to exhale, activate the core, and pull the shoulder blades together and back.

2. Begin to extend the thoracic spine, attempting to move one thoracic vertebra at a time and being careful not to hyperextend the lower back.

3. Hold the top position. Then slowly begin to inhale while lowering the torso back down to the starting position, maintaining the head position and keeping tension on the extensors.

Trainer Techniques

1. Monitor spine and pelvic positioning, thoracic and scapular movement

2. Cue spinal erectors

3. Spot under rib cage

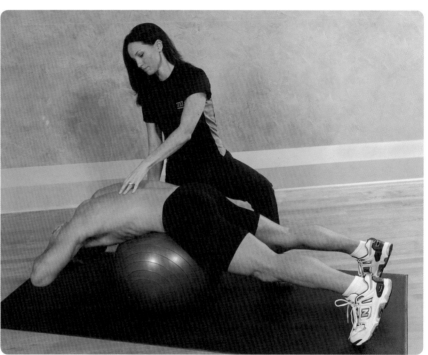

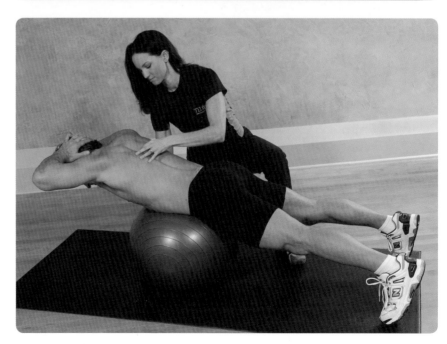

Half Ball Trunk Lateral Flexion

This exercise isolaterally targets the quadratus lumborum, internal obliques, and portions of the external obliques, rectus abdominis, and spinal extensors to the side of movement. Use of the ball can increase the range of motion if beginning in a position of lateral flexion to the opposite side, and it also requires some different core, trunk, and hip musculature recruitment to correct for tilting-response challenges. Variations in the angle and weight load can be made by adjusting the body position on the ball. Depending on the lifter's ability and goals, altering leg position to increase or decrease hip abductor involvement is also a viable option.

Target Muscles

Spinal lateral flexors, quadratus lumborum, internal obliques, ipsilateral spinal flexors, ipsilateral trunk extensors

Joint Motions

Trunk lateral flexion

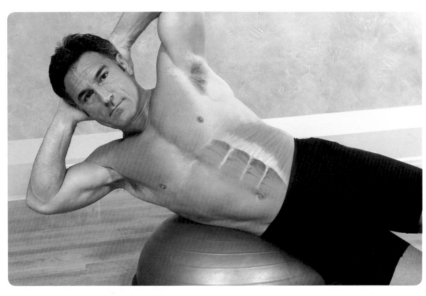

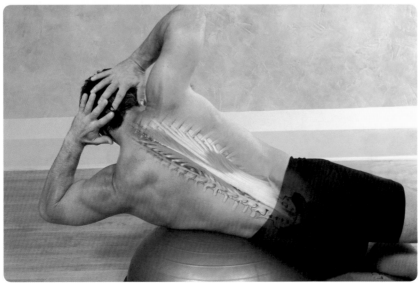

Half Ball Trunk Lateral Flexion

Alignment and Positioning

1. Lie on your side over the half ball, with the bottom leg placed in front of the body and the top leg straight and slightly behind the body.

2. Bend the spine comfortably over the ball, place the bottom arm overhead, and place the top arm against the body or overhead depending on the desired resistance. Begin with a full breath of air.

Motion and Stabilization

1. Slowly begin to exhale, activate the core, and pull the lower ribs toward the crest of the pelvic girdle, attempting to move laterally, one vertebra at a time.

2. Pull the trunk up and over as far as possible without flexing or extending the spine, while continuing to exhale.

3. Hold, then slowly begin to inhale while lowering the torso back down to the starting position, maintaining the head position and keeping tension on the lateral flexors.

Trainer Techniques

1. Monitor spine and pelvic positioning, spine and head movement

2. Cue quadratus lumborum and internal obliques

3. Spot under rib cage or help support head

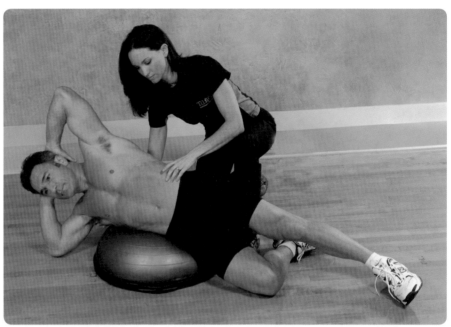

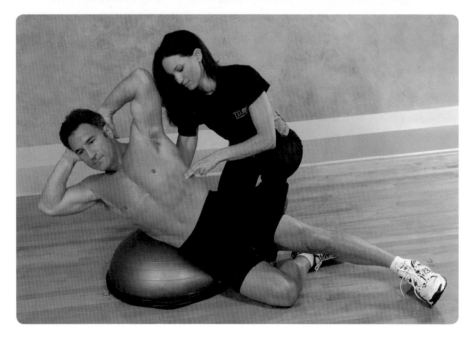

Supine Trunk Rotation

This exercise is designed to begin working on loaded isolated rotation of the spine. It allows the lifter to begin strengthening the external obliques and associated trunk rotators in a stabilized position. The athlete should develop the strength and control of these muscles before progressing to more integrated movements. Once integrated movements are required, the body will use other joints and muscles to compensate for any weakness or lack of movement in spinal rotation.

Target Muscles

Spinal rotators (external oblique, contralateral internal oblique), spinal flexors, transversospinalis group

Joint Motions

Trunk rotation

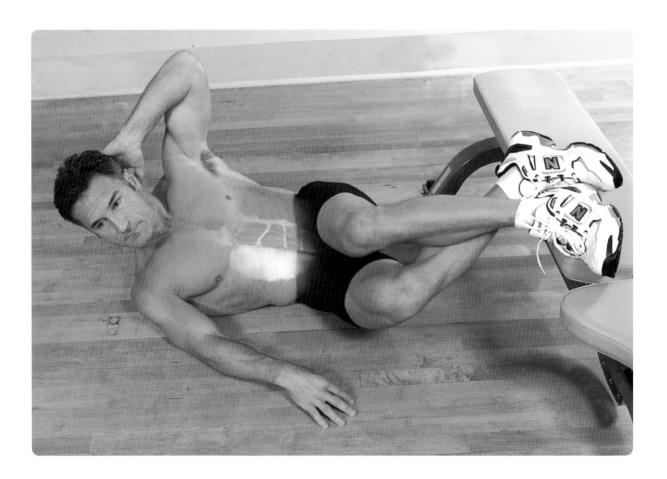

Alignment and Positioning

1. Lie supine on the floor with the feet braced lightly on a low bench or chair.

2. Place one leg over the other. Rotate the pelvis and legs over about 35 to 45 degrees with the sternum still facing up.

3. Place the bottom hand on the side and the other hand behind the head. Begin with the shoulders slightly off the ground and a full breath of air.

Motion and Stabilization

1. Slowly begin to exhale, activate the core, and pull the rib cage slightly up and over to align with the pelvis, keeping the head in a neutral position.

2. Hold the top position while continuing to exhale and contracting the core, abdominal, and oblique muscles.

3. Slowly begin to inhale while lowering the torso back down and over to the starting position, maintaining the head position and keeping tension on the abdominal muscles and obliques.

Trainer Techniques

1. Monitor spine and pelvic positioning, spine and head movement

2. Cue external obliques and abdominals

3. Spot under rib cage or help support head

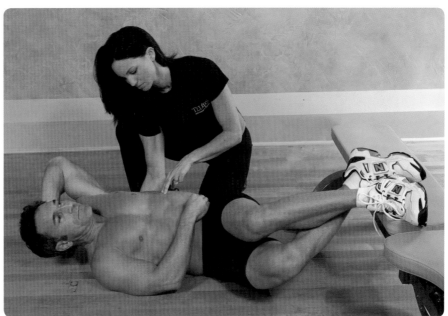

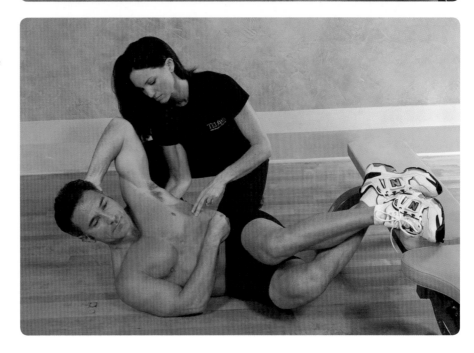

Machine Trunk Rotation

This exercise is designed to strengthen isolated spinal rotation and the anterior oblique subsystem. The use of the machine allows the lifter to develop rotational movement with little stabilization demand, and it provides a brace to anchor the opposite thigh and avoid promoting high levels of hip adductor assistance. This beginning rotational exercise helps to assess and strengthen present active ranges of available spinal rotation before performing more advanced rotational exercises.

Target Muscles

Anterior oblique subsystem (external oblique, contralateral hip adductors, contralateral internal oblique), rectus abdominis, transversospinalis group

Joint Motions

Trunk rotation

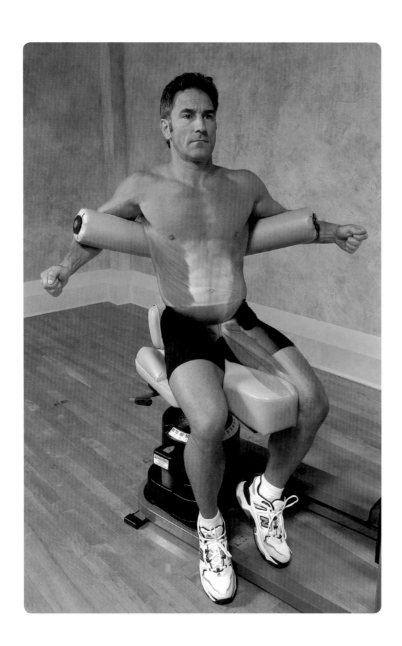

Machine Trunk Rotation

Alignment and Positioning

1. Position the machine to about 45 degrees or the specific amount of spinal rotation desired. Be sure not to set the limit any farther than you can presently actively rotate the spine without resistance!

2. Begin in a rotated position but with good posture and with close to a natural arch in the lower back. Position the arms over the pads and the legs firmly against the pads.

3. Draw a deep breath, allowing the abdominal area to slightly distend with the spine. Avoid any shrugging of the shoulder blades.

Motion and Stabilization

1. Slowly begin to exhale, activate the core, and begin rotating the torso while avoiding flexing or extending the spine.

2. Rotate just slightly past a neutral position (where the torso and pelvis would be directly aligned) while continuing to exhale and contracting the core muscles.

3. Slowly begin to inhale while rotating back to the starting position, allowing the abdominal muscles to slightly distend and keeping the scapula stabilized.

Trainer Techniques

1. Monitor spine and pelvic positioning, spine and head movement

2. Cue external obliques, abdominals, contralateral adductors

3. Spot on machine (assist or resist)

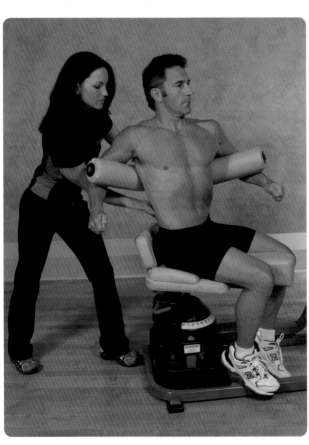
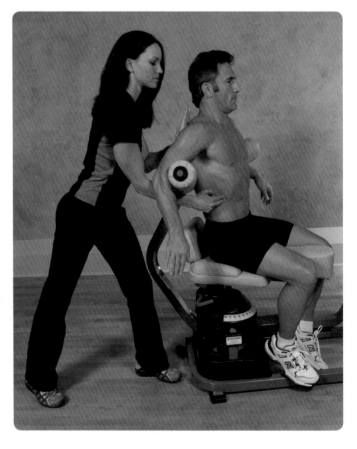

Cable Trunk Rotation With Flexion

This exercise is designed to begin teaching resisted integrated trunk flexion and rotation of the spine. It targets and strengthens the external obliques and associated trunk rotators and flexors while the person is in a standing position that requires lower body musculature for stabilization. This movement pattern would be somewhat transferable to the spinal action involved when throwing a baseball, javelin, or any other object (or even a punch). Teaching and strengthening the body to produce forces in this way should precede faster, more ballistic exercises involving spinal rotation.

Target Muscles

Anterior oblique subsystem (external oblique, contralateral hip adductors, contralateral internal oblique), rectus abdominis, transversospinalis group

Joint Motions

Trunk rotation

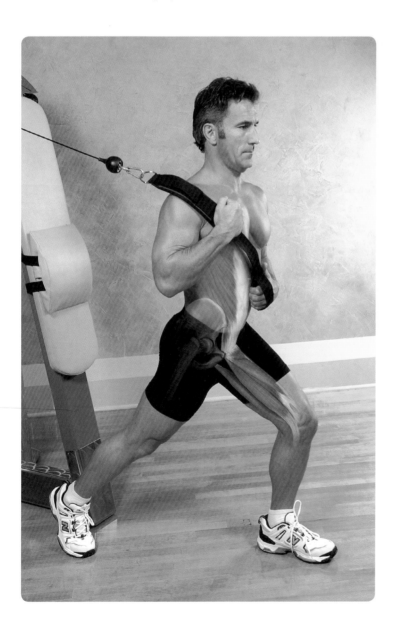

Cable Trunk Rotation With Flexion

Alignment and Positioning

1. Stand in a lunge position, with the back leg straight. Lean the trunk forward, placing the weight over the lead leg while maintaining good posture.

2. Place the strap diagonally over the shoulder and torso opposite to the lead leg.

3. Draw a deep breath, and begin with the trunk in good posture and the pelvis and head squarely aligned.

Motion and Stabilization

1. Slowly begin to exhale. Activate the core while simultaneously flexing and gradually rotating the spine, keeping the pelvis and lower body stabilized.

2. Flex and rotate the spine as far as possible while continuing to exhale and contracting the core muscles.

3. Hold, then slowly begin to inhale while slowly extending and rotating the spine back up to the starting position, maintaining pelvic and leg positioning.

Trainer Techniques

1. Monitor spine and pelvic positioning, spine and head movement

2. Cue external obliques and abdominals

3. Spot back of rib cage or shoulder blade

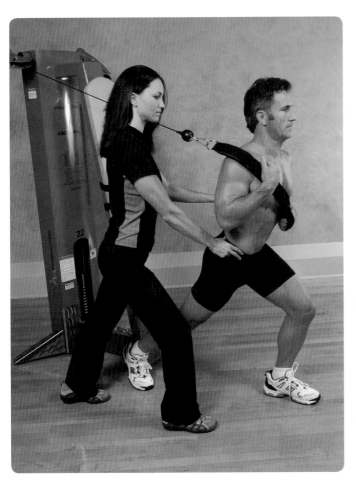 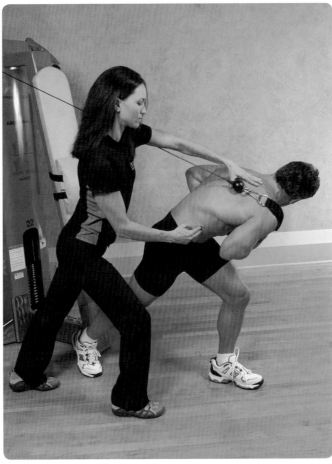

Cable Trunk Rotation With Pull

This exercise is designed to teach integrated and loaded rotation of the spine. It targets and strengthens the external obliques and associated trunk rotators while the person is in a standing position. It also integrates lower body musculature for stabilization and posterior upper body muscles for the pulling movement. Teach the body how to deal with forces in this manner before progressing to faster, more ballistic exercises involving spinal rotation.

Target Muscles

Posterior oblique subsystem (latissimus dorsi, contralateral gluteus maximus, hip external rotators), spinal rotators (external oblique, contralateral internal oblique, transversospinalis group), shoulder and scapular pulling muscles

Joint Motions

Trunk rotation, scapular retraction, shoulder horizontal abduction, elbow flexion

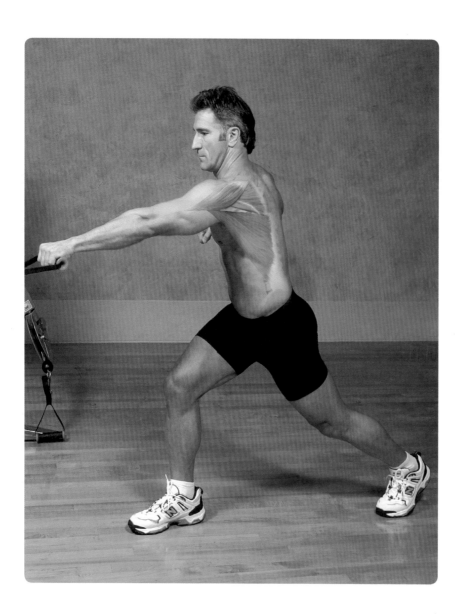

Cable Trunk Rotation With Pull

Alignment and Positioning

1. Stand in a lunge position, with the back leg straight. Lean the trunk forward, placing the weight over the lead leg while maintaining good posture.

2. Grasp the handle with the hand opposite of the lead leg, and begin with the arm straight and perpendicular to the trunk, with the elbow out.

3. Draw a deep breath, and begin with the trunk rotated, keeping the pelvis and head squarely aligned.

Motion and Stabilization

1. Slowly begin to exhale, activate the core, and rotate the spine while pulling the arm out and back, keeping the head and pelvis straight.

2. Rotate the spine and pull the arm back while continuing to exhale and contracting the core muscles.

3. Hold, then slowly begin to inhale while rotating the torso back around and down to the starting position, maintaining the head and pelvic position.

Trainer Techniques

1. Monitor spine and pelvic positioning, spine and head movement

2. Cue lats, posterior delts, and contralateral glutes

3. Spot on wrist, elbow, or rib cage

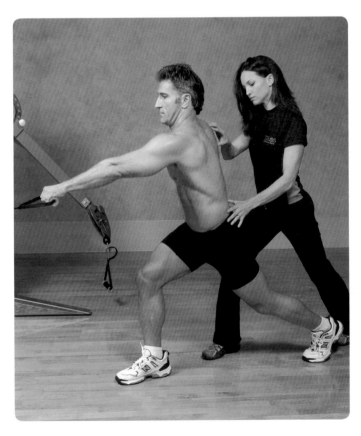
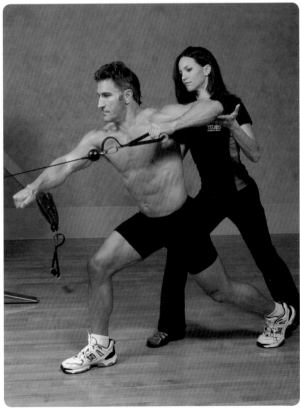

Cable Trunk Rotation With Press

This exercise also teaches how to perform integrated and loaded rotation of the spine. It targets and strengthens the external obliques and associated trunk rotators from a standing position. It also integrates lower body musculature for stabilization and anterior upper body muscles for the pulling movement. Teach the body how to deal with forces in this manner before progressing to faster, more ballistic exercises involving spinal rotation.

Target Muscles

Anterior oblique subsystem (external oblique, contralateral hip adductors, contralateral internal oblique), rectus abdominis, transversospinalis group, shoulder and scapular pushing muscles

Joint Motions

Trunk rotation, scapular protraction, shoulder horizontal adduction, elbow extension

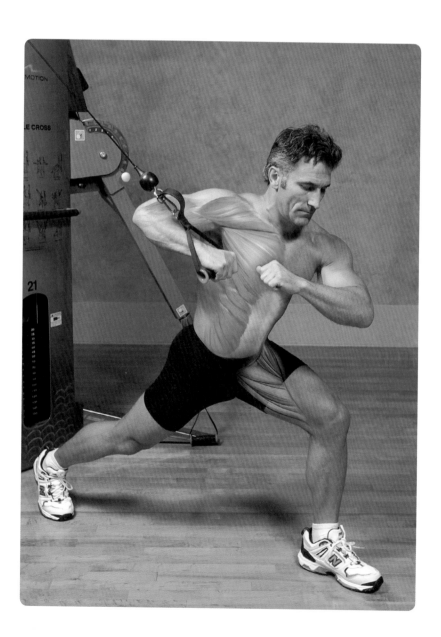

Alignment and Positioning

1. Position the feet on the balance board just outside shoulder width and angled out about 20 to 30 degrees, with the knees and hips slightly flexed.

2. Begin with the hands by the sides, the shoulder blades pulled back, and the spine and head in good posture.

3. Exhale, activate the core, and contract the trunk, hip, and leg muscles to stabilize the starting position.

Motion and Stabilization

1. Slowly begin to inhale, push the hips back, and allow the knees to bend naturally and the trunk to lean forward.

2. Slowly raise the arms for counterbalance, and lower the body until the crest of the pelvis presses against the top of the thigh (or as far as possible) while maintaining proper posture and balance.

3. Hold, then slowly begin to exhale, activate the core, and press the body back up to the starting position while maintaining proper posture and pelvic positioning.

Trainer Techniques

1. Monitor spine and pelvic positioning, hip, knee, and ankle motion

2. Cue glutes and quads

3. Spot under the rib cage

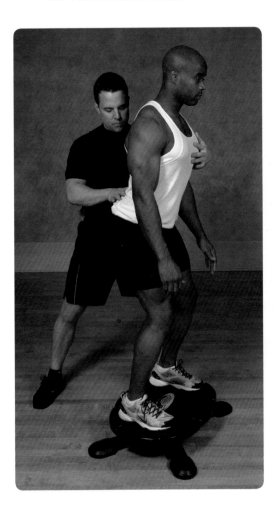

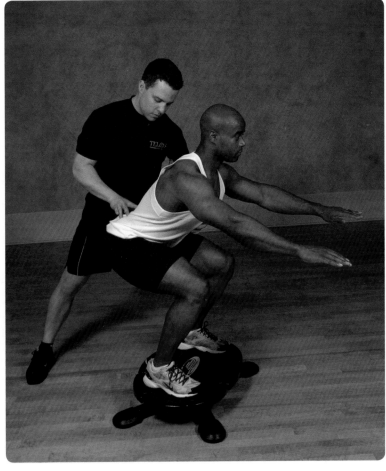

Dumbbell Deadlift (Wide-Stance Squat)

This exercise is performed similarly to any squat movement, but a wider stance is used to allow the dumbbell and the arms to drop between the legs. This exercise targets the hip and knee extensors but also works posterior trunk muscles as stabilizers. It begins loading the squat in a manner very transferable to life demands. Most people must routinely perform this movement pattern in order to pick up a box, a container, or other miscellaneous objects. Heavy loads are difficult to perform with this exercise, because the dumbbell will tend to protract the scapula, which encourages flexion of the thoracic spine and reduces optimal posture.

Target Muscles

Hip extensors (glutes, hamstrings, hip adductors), knee extensors (quadriceps), spinal extensors

Joint Motions

Hip extension, knee extension

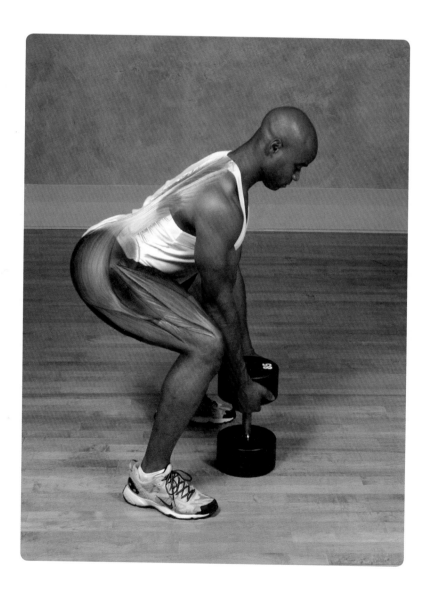

Dumbbell Deadlift (Wide-Stance Squat)

Alignment and Positioning

1. Position the feet well outside shoulder width and angled out about 30 to 45 degrees.

2. Squat and grasp the dumbbell with the arms straight and between the legs.

3. Begin in the squat position, with the hips and knees flexed and the trunk leaned forward in good posture. Draw a deep breath.

Motion and Stabilization

1. Slowly begin to exhale, activate the core, and press the body up by extending the hips and knees while pulling the shoulders back, keeping the dumbbell close to the legs.

2. Hold the top position, continue to exhale, further activate the core, and contract the trunk, hip, and leg muscles to stabilize.

3. Slowly begin to inhale and squat back down, maintaining proper posture and pelvic positioning while lowering the dumbbell down (keeping it close to the legs) until back to the starting position.

Trainer Techniques

1. Monitor spine and pelvic positioning, hip, knee, and ankle motion

2. Cue glutes and quads

3. Spot under the rib cage or on the dumbbell

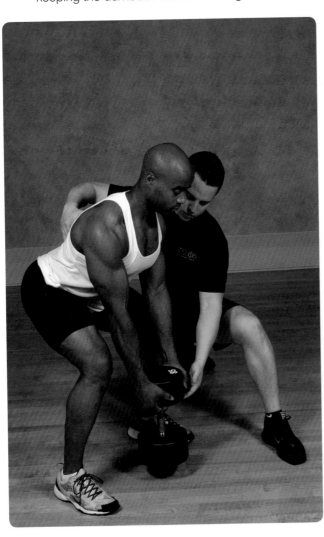
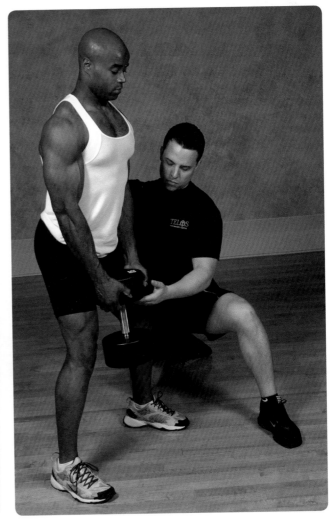

Barbell Deadlift (Narrow-Stance Squat)

This exercise is similar to the traditional deadlift, except a modified starting position is used to reduce lumbar disc compression and lower back strain. All deadlifts are basically a squat movement challenging the hip and knee extensors and including high stabilization demands for the spinal extensors. The Barbell Deadlift utilizes a narrow stance as compared to the Dumbbell Deadlift and again places the load below the body's center of gravity. The deadlift transfers well to life's heavier lifting demands, but loads are limited by grip strength.

Target Muscles

Hip extensors (glutes, hamstrings, hip adductors), knee extensors (quadriceps), spinal extensors

Joint Motions

Hip extension, knee extension

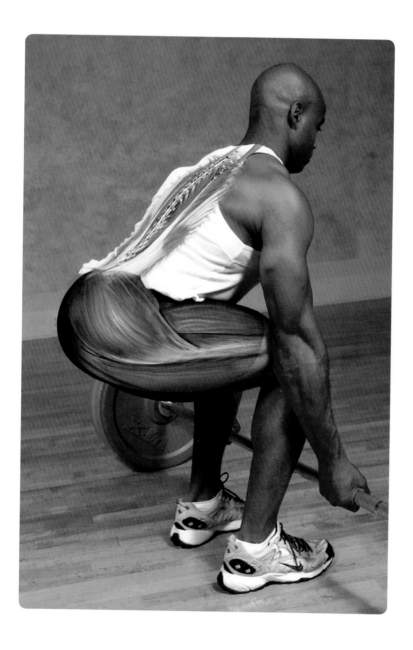

Barbell Deadlift (Narrow-Stance Squat)

Alignment and Positioning

1. Set the barbell at the appropriate height to allow for the ability to maintain the natural lumbar curve and good posture.

2. Position the feet just inside shoulder width and pointed straight ahead. Grip the bar with a shoulder-width, alternate grip.

3. Begin in a squat position, with the hips and knees flexed and the trunk leaned forward in good posture. Draw a deep breath.

Motion and Stabilization

1. Slowly begin to exhale, activate the core, and press the body up by extending the hips and knees while pulling the shoulders back, keeping the bar close to the legs.

2. Hold the top position, continue to exhale, further activate the core, and contract the trunk, hip, and leg muscles to stabilize.

3. Slowly begin to inhale and squat back down, maintaining proper posture and pelvic positioning while lowering the bar down (keeping it close to the legs) until back to the starting position.

Trainer Techniques

1. Monitor spine and pelvic positioning, hip, knee, and ankle motion

2. Cue glutes and quads

3. Spot under the rib cage

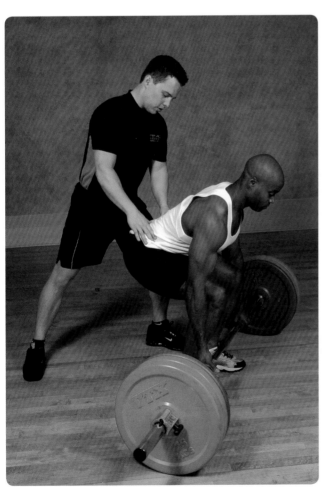 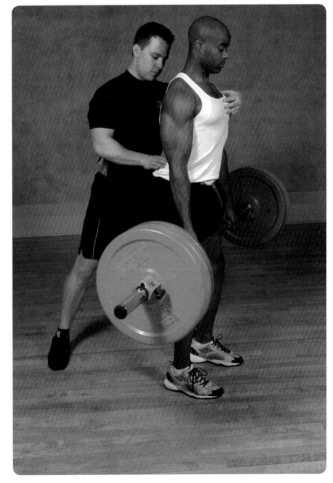

Barbell Squat

This exercise maximally loads the squat movement and targets the hip and knee extensors. Bar placement on the upper back with the scapula retracted helps to stabilize the thoracic spine in an extended position, making posture easier to maintain under heavy loads and during long sets. In life, people may rarely place large loads on their backs to lift them, but all squats are considered general movement pattern training that transfers better to life demands than many other leg exercises. For individuals with neck, shoulder, and spinal stability concerns you may need to consider other squat exercises.

Target Muscles

Hip extensors (glutes, hamstrings, hip adductors), knee extensors (quadriceps), spinal extensors

Joint Motions

Hip extension, knee extension

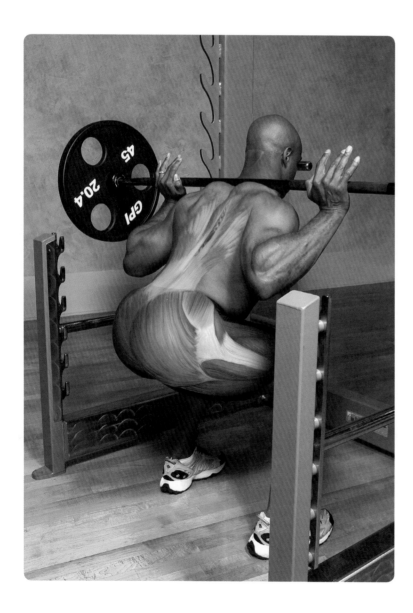

Alignment and Positioning

1. Place the barbell just above the scapula, with the hands placed comfortably on the bar and the elbows pointed down.

2. Position the feet just outside shoulder width and angled out about 20 to 30 degrees, with the knees and hips slightly flexed and the spine and head held in good posture.

3. Exhale, activate the core, and contract the trunk, hip, and leg muscles to stabilize the starting position.

Motion and Stabilization

1. Slowly begin to inhale, push the hips back, and allow the knees to bend naturally and the trunk to lean forward.

2. Lower the body until the crest of the pelvis presses against the top of the thigh (or as far as possible) while maintaining proper posture.

3. Hold, then slowly begin to exhale, activate the core, and press the body and barbell back up to the starting position while maintaining proper posture and pelvic positioning.

Trainer Techniques

1. Monitor spine and pelvic positioning, hip, knee, and ankle motion

2. Cue glutes and quads

3. Spot under the rib cage

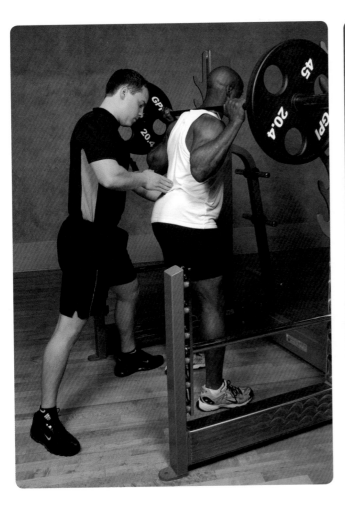

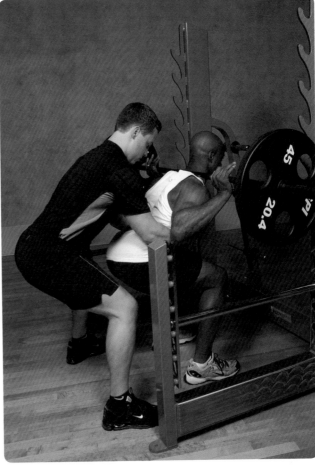

Machine Seated Leg Press

This exercise is good for targeting and strengthening the hip and knee extensors. Though not as transferable as a squat, leg pressing exercises may prove helpful for hypertrophy goals simply by adding more compound leg movement to a program. Small variations in feet positioning can be selected to better emphasize hip or knee extensor contribution. However, it is important to maintain the knee alignment and pelvic-spinal positioning described on page 151 to avoid additional risk of wear or injury to the knees or lower back area.

Target Muscles

Hip extensors (glutes, hamstrings, hip adductors), knee extensors (quadriceps)

Joint Motions

Hip extension, knee extension

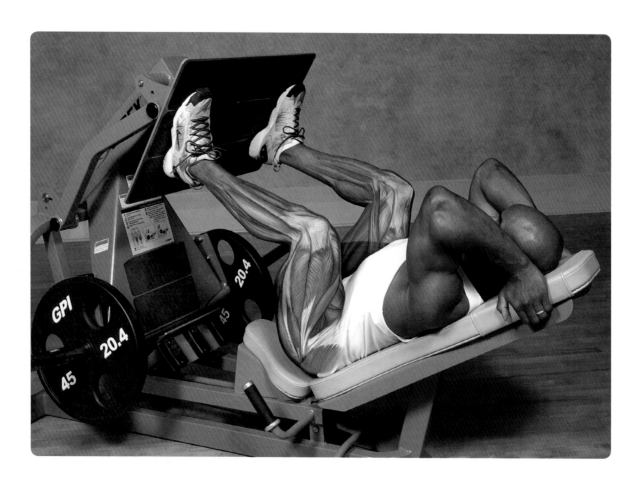

Alignment and Positioning

1. Position the back pad and the feet in a manner that allows you to maintain an arch in the lower back and also prohibits the knees from passing too far over the toes.

2. For a wide stance, position the feet just outside shoulder width and angled out about 20 to 30 degrees. For a narrow stance, the feet should be at hip width and positioned straight.

3. Begin with a slight bend in the hips and knees, a natural arch in the lower back, and the core activated.

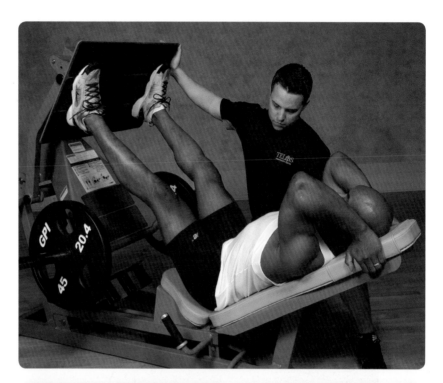

Motion and Stabilization

1. Slowly begin to inhale, and allow the legs and platform to lower until the thigh presses against the crest of the pelvis while maintaining the natural arch in the lower spine.

2. Hold, slowly begin to exhale, activate the core, and press the platform back to the starting position while maintaining the pelvic-spinal positioning described above.

3. Hold and stabilize the starting position; continue to maintain proper pelvic-spinal positioning and bend the knees slightly to avoid resting.

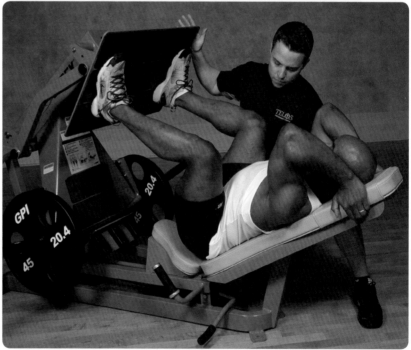

Trainer Techniques

1. Monitor spine and pelvic positioning, hip, knee, and ankle motion

2. Cue glutes and quads

3. Spot on the foot plate (assist or resist)

Body Weight Stationary Lunge

This exercise is good for beginning to strengthen the lunge movement. Lunges are similar to a single-leg squat, so they should be integrated into a program only after the squat has been mastered. This movement prepares the hip and leg muscles to stabilize and lift the body from an asymmetrical position. Such positions produce a torque on the pelvis, which brings additional hip, core, and trunk musculature into play to stabilize the body. The knee and MTP joints (joints of the toes) of the trail leg are also not in the best position to accept higher amounts of load, so positioning of the trunk, pelvis, and back leg is critical.

Target Muscles

Lead leg—hip extensors (glutes, hamstrings, hip adductors), knee extensors (quadriceps)

Joint Motions

Lead leg—hip extension, knee extension

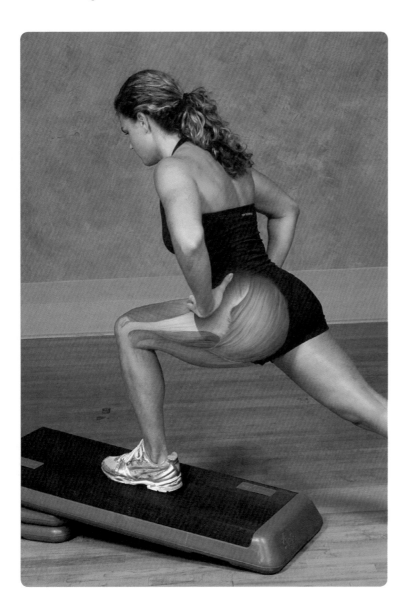

Body Weight Stationary Lunge

Alignment and Positioning

1. Position the legs in a lunge position, with the lead leg far enough out to allow for the desired range of motion.

2. Straighten the back knee and lean forward so that the trunk is in line with the back leg while maintaining proper posture.

3. Begin with a slight bend in the lead hip and knee, a natural arch in the lower back, and the core activated.

Motion and Stabilization

1. Slowly begin to inhale, and allow the trunk to come forward and down until the crest of the pelvis presses against the top of the thigh (or as far as possible) while maintaining proper posture.

2. Be sure to keep the forward knee aligned straight with the toes, without letting it pass too far in front of the toes. Keep the trunk aligned with the back leg.

3. Hold, slowly begin to exhale, activate the core, and with the weight toward the heel, press the body back up to the starting position while maintaining good pelvic-spinal positioning.

Trainer Techniques

1. Monitor spine and pelvic positioning, hip, knee, and ankle motion

2. Cue glutes and quads

3. Spot under the rib cage

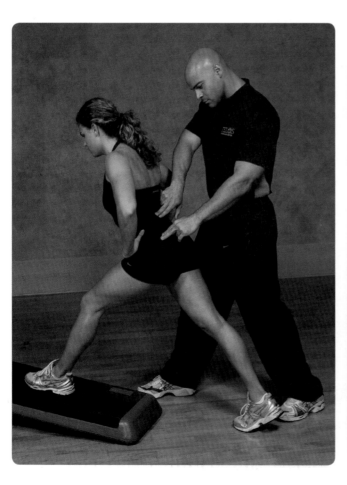
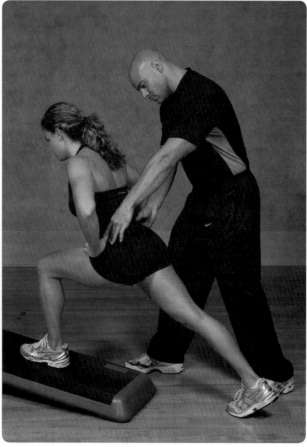

Dumbbell Reverse Lunge

This exercise progresses the lunge from a stationary movement to a more dynamic movement. Since the lifter will be required to stabilize a single-leg position at certain points of the movement, this exercise will place a higher demand on the hip abductors as well as targeting the hip and knee extensors of the lead leg. Use of heavier dumbbells is difficult because they tend to protract the scapula and flex the thoracic spine, diminishing optimal posture. The use of a step (stair) is not necessary but can help to increase range of motion without having to step back as far.

Target Muscles

Lead leg—hip extensors (glutes, hamstrings, hip adductors), knee extensors (quadriceps), hip abductors

Joint Motions

Lead leg—hip extension, knee extension

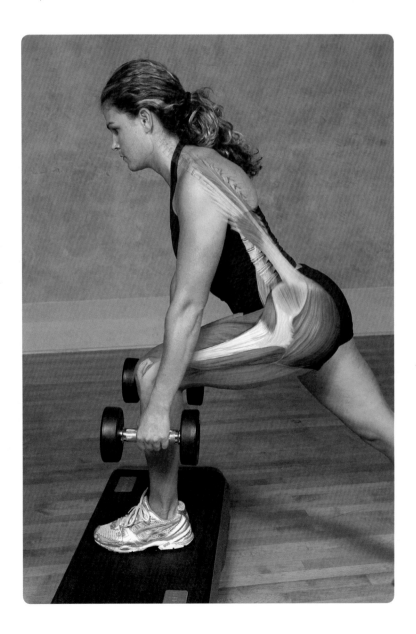

Dumbbell Reverse Lunge

Alignment and Positioning

1. Stand on a small step with most of your weight shifted to the lead leg, with the toe of the other leg just touching the step for balance.

2. Position the trunk in good posture, activate the core, and begin with the arms at the sides.

3. Begin with a slight bend in the knee and hip of the lead leg, a natural arch in the lower back, and the core activated.

Motion and Stabilization

1. Begin to inhale, step back off the step, and lower the body so that the crest of the pelvis touches the top of the thigh of the lead leg, while keeping good posture.

2. Be sure to keep the forward knee aligned straight with the toes, without letting it pass too far in front of the toes. Keep the trunk aligned with the straight back leg.

3. Hold, slowly begin to exhale, activate the core, and with the weight toward the heel, press the body back up to the starting position while maintaining proper pelvic-spinal positioning.

Trainer Techniques

1. Monitor spine and pelvic positioning, hip, knee, and ankle motion

2. Cue glutes and quads

3. Spot under the rib cage

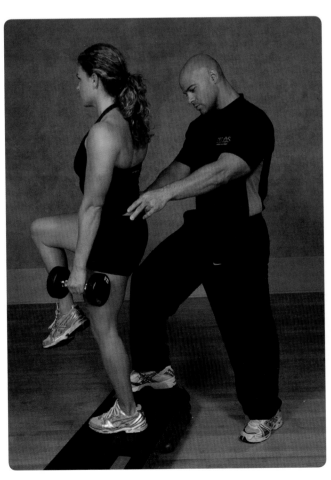
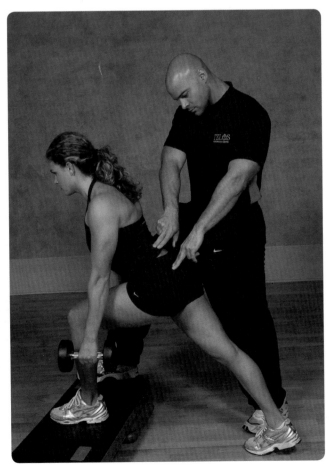

Dumbbell Side Lunge

This exercise is simply a reverse lunge performed with a more lateral or diagonal movement. This increased lateral movement will demand more hip adductor recruitment to assist the hip and knee extensors of the lead leg. Use of heavier dumbbells tends to protract the scapula and flex the thoracic spine, diminishing optimal posture. The use of a step (stair) is not necessary but can help to increase range of motion without having to step as far back or out.

Target Muscles

Lead leg—hip extensors (glutes, hamstrings, hip adductors), knee extensors (quadriceps), hip abductors

Joint Motions

Lead leg—hip extension, knee extension

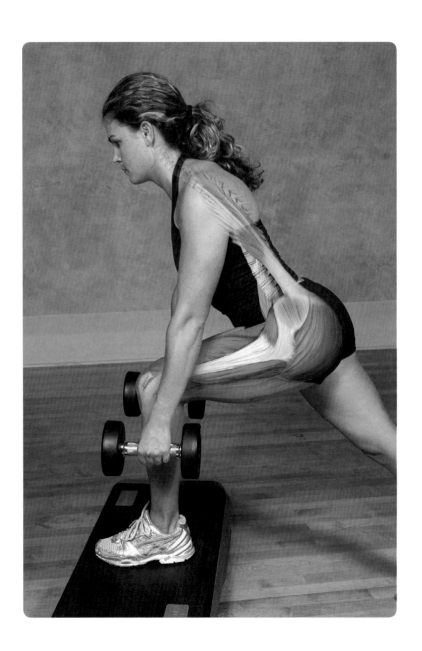

Alignment and Positioning

1. Stand on a small step with the lead foot and knee angled out about 20 to 30 degrees and the opposite foot just touching the step for balance.

2. Position the trunk in good posture, activate the core, and begin with the weighted arm slightly in front of the body.

3. Begin with a slight bend in the knee and hip of the lead leg, and with a natural arch in the lower back.

Motion and Stabilization

1. Begin to inhale, step off the step at a diagonal angle, and lower the body to a point where the crest of the pelvis presses against the top of the thigh of the lead leg, while maintaining good posture.

2. Be sure to keep the lead knee aligned straight with the toes, without letting it pass too far in front of the toes. Keep the trunk aligned with the straight back leg.

3. Hold, slowly begin to exhale, activate the core, and with the weight toward the heel, press the body back up to the starting position while maintaining proper posture.

Trainer Techniques

1. Monitor spine and pelvic positioning, hip, knee, and ankle motion

2. Cue glutes and quads

3. Spot under the rib cage

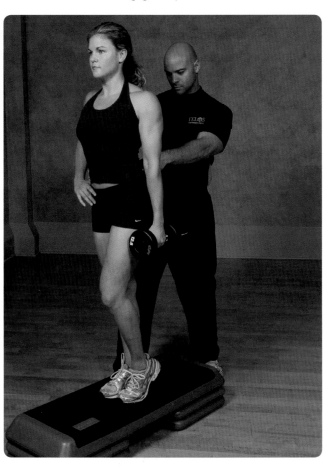
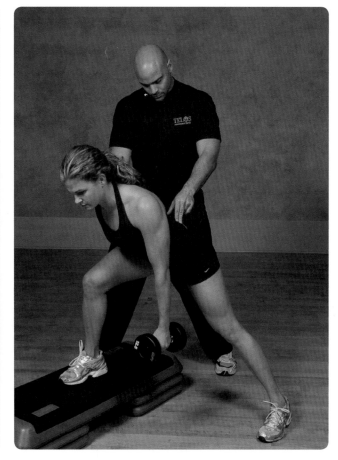

Med Ball Traveling Lunge (Side Load)

This exercise further increases the balance and stability challenges because the movement is far more dynamic than a stationary or reverse lunge. The Med Ball is used for added resistance and may be more comfortable than using plates or dumbbells. The ball may be placed in front for a balanced anterior challenge, or to the side for an unbalanced lateral challenge. For heavier posterior loads, a barbell would probably work best. Choose the appropriate level and placement of loads to match the lifter's current abilities and specific goals. Typically, only light to moderate loads are needed for any traveling lunge because maximum strength development is not an appropriate goal for this exercise.

Target Muscles

Lead leg—hip extensors (glutes, hamstrings, hip adductors), knee extensors (quadriceps), hip abductors

Joint Motions

Lead leg—hip extension, knee extension

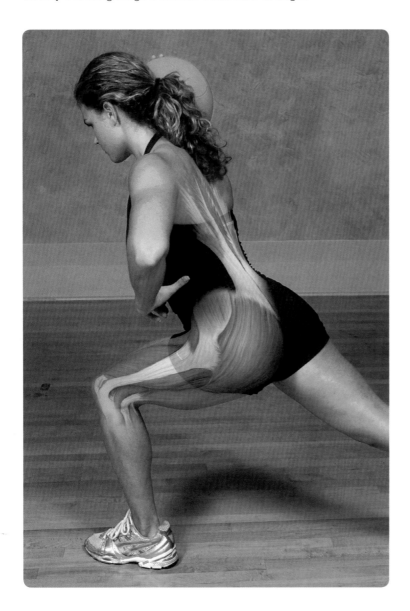

Med Ball Traveling Lunge (Side Load)

Alignment and Positioning

1. Stand with your weight on the lead leg and with the toes of the other leg just touching the ground for balance.

2. Position the ball on the shoulder, with the trunk in good posture. Activate the core and begin with a slight bend in the knee and hip of the lead leg.

Motion and Stabilization

1. Begin to inhale, lunge forward, and lean the trunk until the crest of the pelvis touches the top of the thigh of the lead leg (or as far as comfortable for the desired range of motion).

2. Be sure to keep the forward knee aligned straight with the toes, without letting it pass too far in front of the toes. Keep the trunk aligned with the straight back leg.

3. Hold, slowly begin to exhale, activate the core, and with the weight toward the heel, press the body forward and up to the starting position while maintaining proper posture. Repeat with the same leg or alternate if desired.

Trainer Techniques

1. Monitor spine and pelvic positioning, hip, knee, and ankle motion

2. Cue glutes and quads

3. Spot under the rib cage

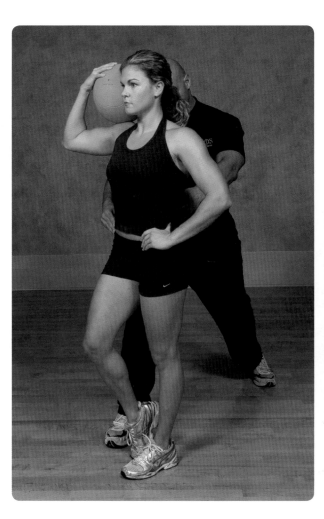
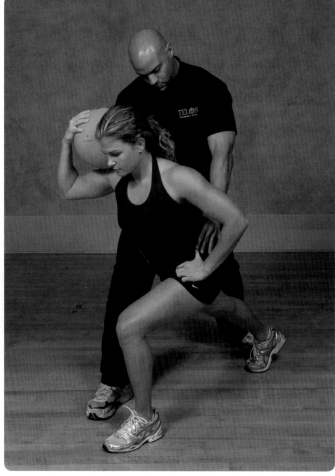

Barbell Hang Clean

This exercise is not designed for targeting muscles to achieve any aesthetic-based goal, but rather it is often selected for certain performance-based goals, such as improving plyometric actions of the hip and leg muscles and increasing combined lower body and trunk power. This movement requires a fast tempo or lifting speed and specific timing of various joint mechanics in order to obtain the desired benefits and reduce associated risks. Careful attention to technique and goal-to-risk assessment should be done before selecting this exercise or prescribing loads and volume.

Target Muscles

Ankle-knee-hip-trunk extensor chain, upper and mid trapezius, levator scapula

Joint Motions

Ankle extension, knee extension, hip extension, slight spinal extension, scapular elevation and retraction, shoulder abduction, shoulder external rotation

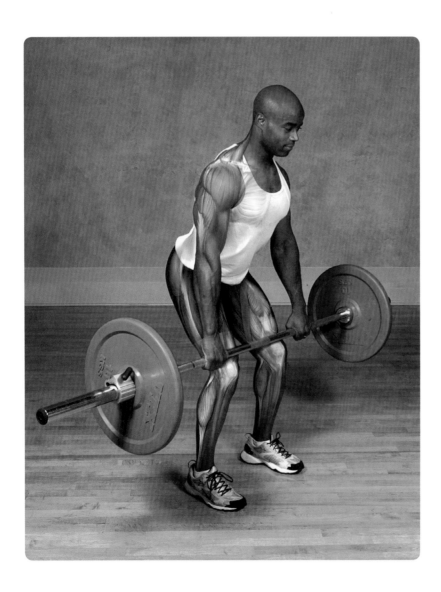

Alignment and Positioning

1. Stand in good posture with the feet directly under the hips. Grasp the bar with an overhand grip, with the hands just outside shoulder-width apart.

2. Flex the hips and knees slightly to position the spine at an approximate 45-degree angle, with good posture and the bar close to the thighs. Draw a deep breath.

Motion and Stabilization

1. Quickly drop to a shallow squat, then immediately activate the core and quickly press off the ground with a jumping movement while pulling the shoulder blades and bar up.

2. Continue to extend the ankles, knees, and hips until the body is almost or just off the ground while continuing to pull the bar up to about chin level.

3. Quickly drop down under the bar while rotating the elbows and relaxing the wrists to catch the bar on the upper chest. Then front squat the weight to an upright position.

4. Quickly but cautiously flip the bar down to the starting position.

Trainer Techniques

1. Monitor spine and pelvic positioning
2. Coach technique
3. Spot behind and to the side

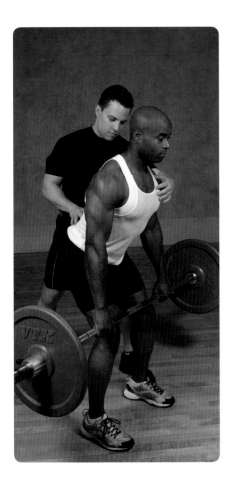
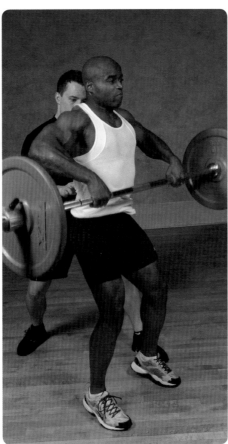
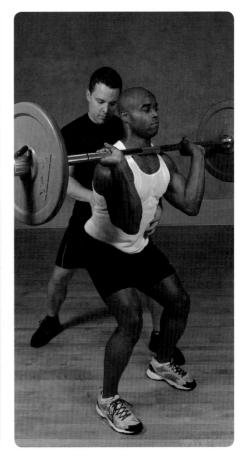

Dumbbell Snatch

This exercise is not designed for targeting muscles, but rather for targeting a movement to achieve specific performance-based goals. This exercise helps to improve plyometric actions of the hip and leg muscles and increases lower body and trunk extension power. This movement requires a fast tempo or lifting speed and specific timing of various joint mechanics in order to obtain the desired benefits and reduce associated risks. Careful attention to technique and goal-to-risk assessment should be done before selecting this exercise or prescribing loads and volume.

Target Muscles

Ankle-knee-hip-trunk extensor chain, shoulder flexors, scapular elevators, shoulder stabilizers

Joint Motions

Ankle extension, knee extension, hip extension, slight spinal extension, scapular elevation and retraction, shoulder flexion, shoulder external rotation

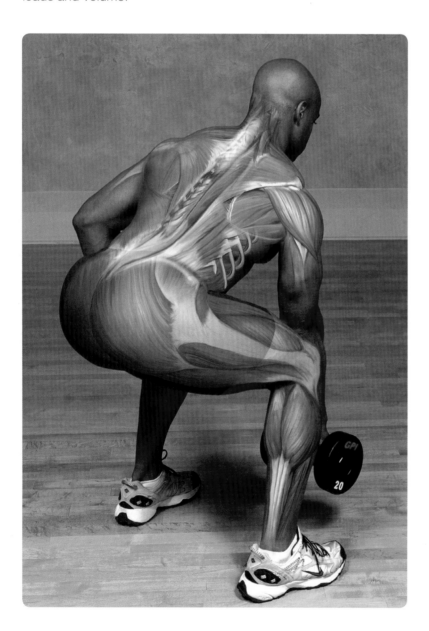

Alignment and Positioning

1. Brace the body on a hanging or Roman chair, with good posture, the elbows securely positioned under the shoulders, the scapula depressed, and the sacrum braced against the pad.

2. Begin with a full breath of air and with one leg positioned straight and just in front of the hips to create slight tension on the abdominal muscles. The other leg is bent so the thigh is about parallel to the ground.

Motion and Stabilization

1. Slowly begin to exhale, and activate the core muscles while raising the straight leg, keeping the knee locked and the ankle flexed back.

2. Continue to pull the leg up as high as possible. Then hold at the top position while maintaining proper posture and continuing to exhale and contract the core muscles and hip flexors.

3. Slowly begin to inhale, and lower the leg back down to the starting position while maintaining posture. Then repeat with the same leg or alternate with the other leg.

Trainer Techniques

1. Monitor lumbar spine and pelvic positioning, hip motion

2. Cue hip flexors, abdominals

3. Spot under the leg

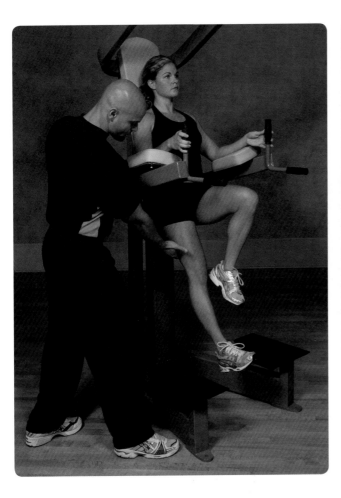
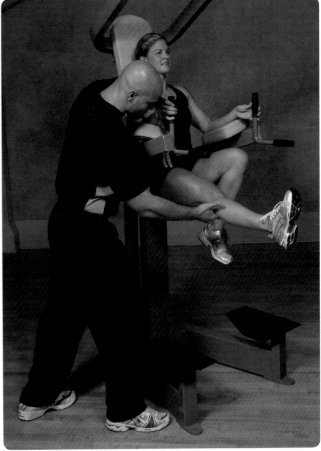

Swiss Ball Double-Leg Hip Flexion

This exercise targets strengthening the hip flexor musculature, and it also increases the challenge for the abdominal muscles and neck flexors. Using the Swiss ball places increased demand on the core and trunk muscles for balancing and stabilization. Single-leg and bent-knee versions should be suggested before lifters attempt the double-leg option. Increased loads can be implemented by simply adjusting the body farther out on the ball. Neck flexor strength is a prerequisite for this exercise, because the head cannot easily be rested at any time during the movement.

Target Muscles

Hip flexors (psoas, iliacus, rectus femoris), core, spinal flexors

Joint Motions

Hip flexion

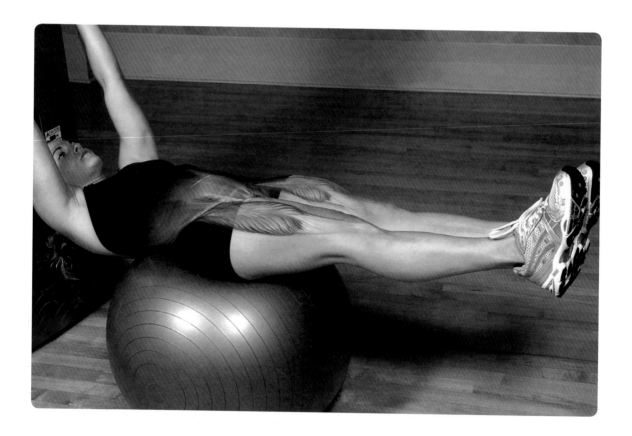

Swiss Ball Double-Leg Hip Flexion

Alignment and Positioning

1. Lie supine on a Swiss ball, with good posture and the hands anchored on a stable object.

2. Begin with both legs up and straight, and with the ankles flexed.

3. Begin with the head and spine in good posture and the chin slightly tucked. Contract the core, abdominal, and hip flexor muscles.

Motion and Stabilization

1. Slowly begin to inhale, and lower the legs until the thighs are parallel with the body (or as low as possible) while maintaining posture and head position.

2. Hold at the bottom position, then slowly begin to exhale, activate the core, and pull the legs up to the starting position while maintaining head and spinal position.

3. Hold again at the top position, maintaining the straight leg and spinal positioning to actively stretch the hamstrings and calves while further contracting the core muscles. Then slowly inhale and repeat.

Trainer Techniques

1. Monitor lumbar spine and pelvic positioning, hip motion

2. Cue hip flexors, abdominals

3. Spot under the leg, possibly support under back of head

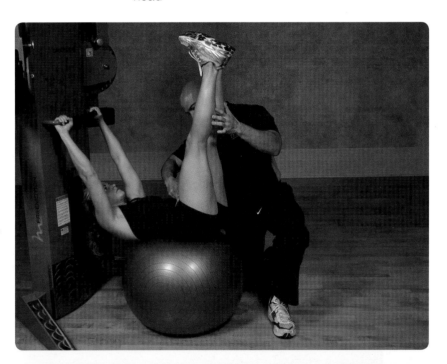

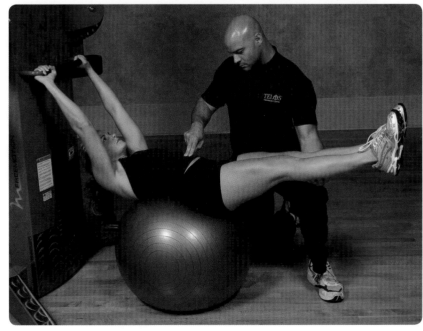

45-Degree Hip Extension

This exercise is designed to target the glutes and hamstring musculature and will also work the spinal erectors as stabilizers. Slight external rotation of the hips is presented on this exercise to further target the glutes but is not necessary or always advisable. Due to the knee being forced into a "locked position," people with knee concerns, larger people, or people with goals that require use of heavy additional loads may find that barbell and dumbbell hip extension exercises are better options.

Target Muscles

Hip extensors (glutes, hamstrings), spinal extensors, core

Joint Motions

Hip extension

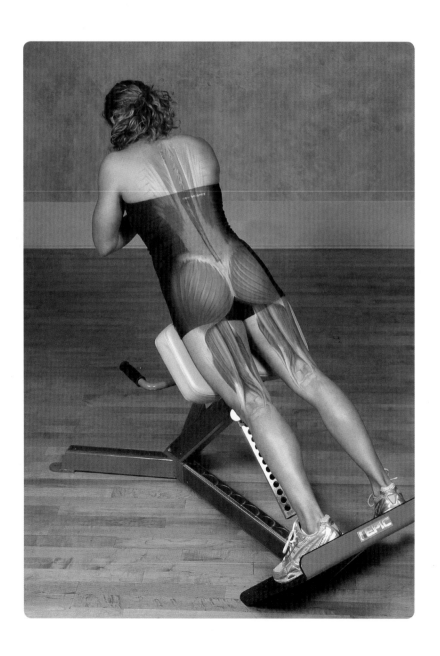

45-Degree Hip Extension

Alignment and Positioning

1. Position the brace so that the iliac spine of the pelvis will move freely over the pad. Then stand with the hips and feet straight and slightly externally rotated (about 30 degrees).

2. Retract the scapula and pull the arms slightly behind the torso, with the spine and head in good posture. (The arms may also be placed across the chest, behind the head, or overhead to further increase the load.)

3. Exhale, activate the core and abdominal muscles, and contract the glutes and hamstrings to stabilize the starting position.

Motion and Stabilization

1. Slowly begin to inhale, and lower the trunk as far as the hamstrings will allow while maintaining proper posture and head position.

2. Hold, slowly begin to exhale, activate the core, and pull the torso back up to the starting position by contracting the glutes and hamstrings. Continue to maintain head and spinal position.

3. Hold and stabilize this position, and finish exhaling while further contracting the core, glutes, and hamstrings.

Trainer Techniques

1. Monitor spine, pelvic, and knee positioning, hip motion

2. Cue glutes, hamstrings

3. Spot under the rib cage

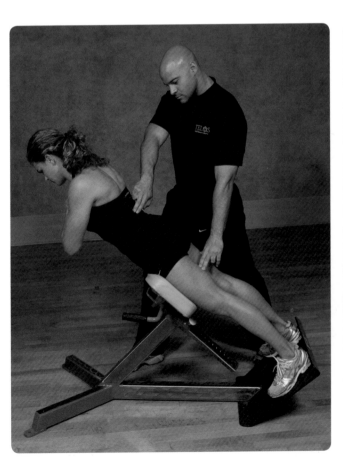

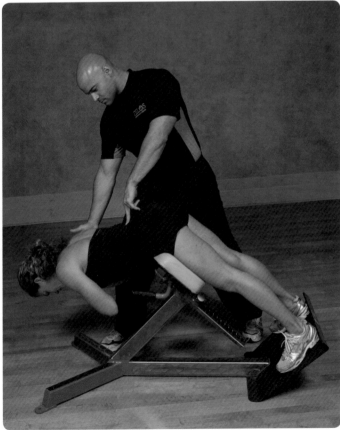

Barbell Hip Extension

This exercise is designed to strengthen the glutes and hamstrings and will also train the spinal erectors as stabilizers. Using barbells, dumbbells, or other free weight loads in unsupported and standing positions allows the lifter to better load the exercise with less risk to the knees as compared to the 45-degree or other machine options. This lifting movement is also very transferable to life demands and can be considered a modified squat movement.

Target Muscles

Hip extensors (glutes, hamstrings), spinal extensors, core

Joint Motions

Hip extension

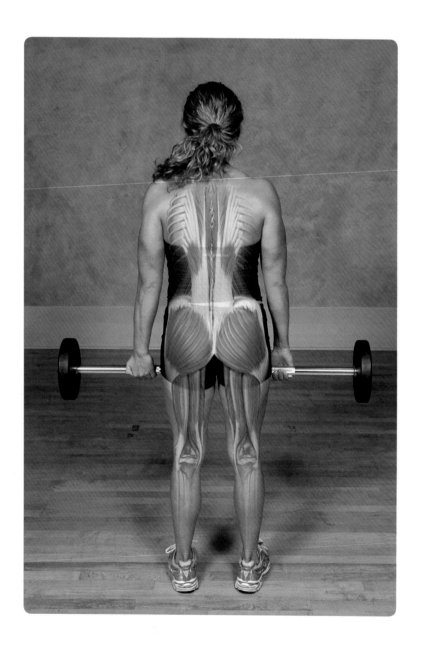

Alignment and Positioning

1. Position the feet straight ahead and directly under the hips, with the knees slightly bent.

2. Place the hands on the bar with an alternate grip, shoulder-width apart. Squat the bar up to the starting position, with the spine in good posture.

3. Begin from a standing position with the shoulders back and the spine and head in good posture. Exhale and activate the core to stabilize the starting position.

Motion and Stabilization

1. Slowly begin to inhale. Push the hips back and lower the trunk as low as the hamstrings will allow while maintaining proper posture and keeping the bar close to the body.

2. Hold at the bottom position. Then slowly begin to exhale, activate the core, and pull the torso back up to the starting position using the glutes and hamstrings while relaxing the arms and maintaining proper posture.

3. Hold and stabilize this position, and finish exhaling while further contracting the core, glutes, and hamstrings.

Trainer Techniques

1. Monitor spine, pelvic, and knee positioning, hip motion

2. Cue glutes, hamstrings

3. Spot under the rib cage or possibly on bar

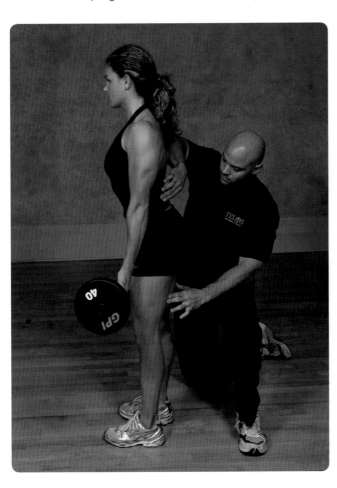
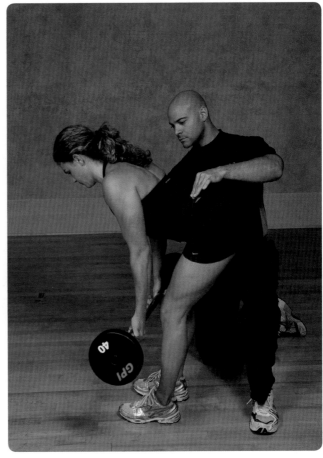

Dumbbell One-Leg Hip Extension

This exercise is designed not only to strengthen the glutes and hamstring musculature but also to train body-righting reflex actions and improve balance. Additional hip and ankle stabilizers of the stationary leg are also highly challenged with this exercise, along with the entire chain of spinal extensor muscles. This exercise is an advanced movement that targets the entire deep longitudinal subsystem. Individuals with limited hip mobility, tight hamstrings, ankle or spinal instability, or poor balance may initially need external assistance for this movement or may require another exercise altogether.

Target Muscles

Hip extensors (glutes, hamstrings), deep longitudinal subsystem (tibialis muscles, peroneus muscles, biceps femoris, sacrotuberal, ligament, spinal extensors), core

Joint Motions

Hip extension

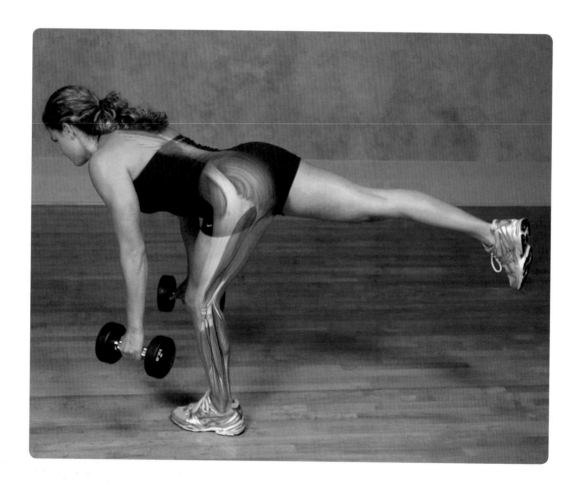

Dumbbell One-Leg Hip Extension

Alignment and Positioning

1. Position the foot of the stationary leg straight ahead, and hold the other leg forward and up in a bent-knee position.

2. Hold the dumbbells relaxed at the sides of the body. Balance and create good posture.

3. Begin with the shoulders back and the spine and head in good posture. Exhale and activate the core.

Motion and Stabilization

1. Slowly begin to inhale, and lower the leg down and back to straighten it while leaning the upper body over as far as the hamstrings will allow. Let the dumbbells lower, keeping them close to the body.

2. Continue to lean over and straighten the back leg while focusing on maintaining optimal posture and a level pelvic position.

3. Hold and balance. Then slowly begin to exhale, activate the core, and pull the leg and torso back up to the starting position using the glutes and hamstrings while maintaining proper posture.

Trainer Techniques

1. Monitor spine, pelvic, knee, and ankle positioning, hip motion

2. Cue glutes, hamstrings

3. Spot under the rib cage or possibly under back leg

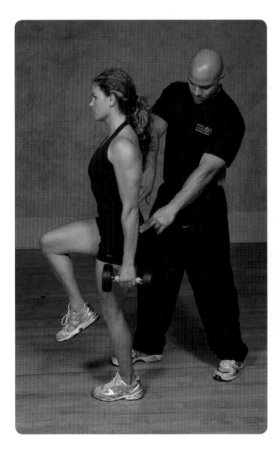
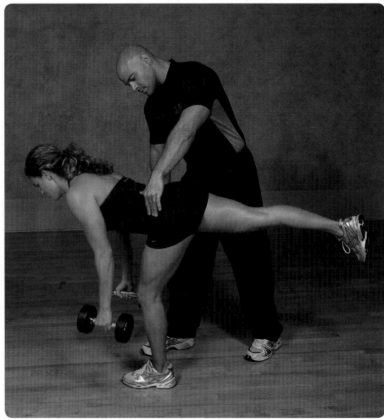

Cable Hip Abduction

This exercise targets the gluteus medius and associated hip abductors. Hip abductors are important for pelvic stability, particularly when standing on one leg or for any walking, lunging, or running movements. Optimal gait performance and one-leg standing exercises rely on prior adequate hip abductor strength that may be best developed initially in an isolated manner, such as that presented with this exercise. Internal and external hip rotation may be added to better target specific regions of the hip abductors.

Target Muscles

Lateral subsystem (hip abductors—gluteus medius, gluteus minimus, tensor fascia latae; contralateral lateral trunk flexors—quadratus lumborum, internal obliques), core

Joint Motions

Hip abduction

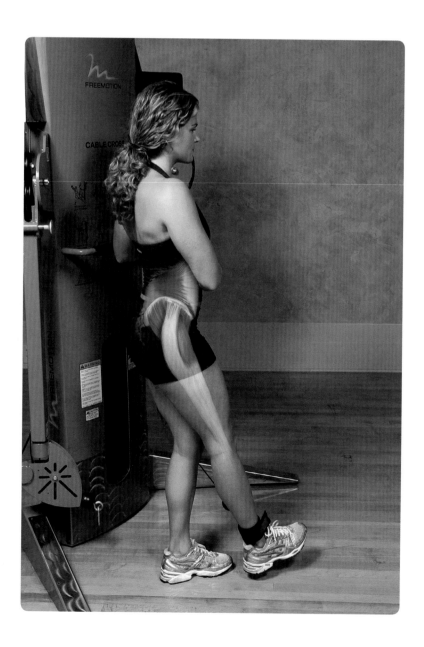

Alignment and Positioning

1. Strap one cable to the outside ankle, and stand with the opposite foot straight ahead and the knee slightly bent.

2. Position the outside leg slightly across the body and in front of the stationary leg, and place the opposite hand lightly on the bar for balance assistance.

3. Begin with the shoulders back, the spine and head in good posture, and the pelvis level. Draw a deep breath.

Motion and Stabilization

1. Slowly begin to exhale, activate the core, and pull the leg across and out from the body while maintaining proper posture and pelvic position.

2. Hold this position and continue to contract the core, trunk, and hip abductors.

3. Slowly begin to inhale, and allow the leg to be pulled back to the starting position while maintaining proper posture and pelvic positioning.

Trainer Techniques

1. Monitor spine, pelvic, knee, and ankle positioning, hip motion

2. Cue hip abductors (both legs)

3. Spot on lower leg

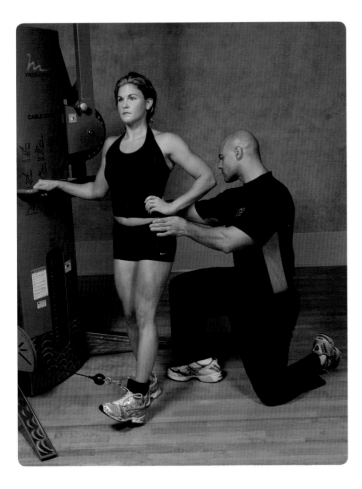 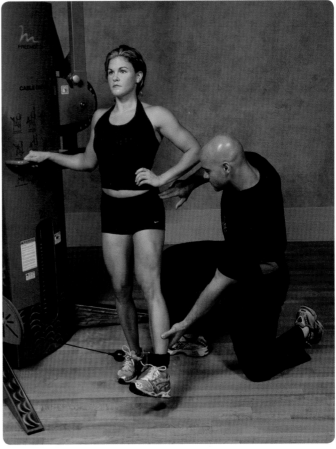

Cable Hip Adduction

The hip adductors not only perform adduction but are also important synergists for hip extension and hip flexion. As such, these versatile muscles are also worked during any squatting or leg pressing movement as well as on certain hip flexion exercises. Therefore, the need for prior or additional isolated strengthening exercises for the hip adductors is not as great as for the hip abductors. However, this exercise may be valuable for specific rehabilitation or performance-related goals.

Target Muscles

Hip adductors (adductor magnus, adductor longus, adductor brevis, pectineus, gracilis), core, anterior oblique subsystem

Joint Motions

Hip adduction

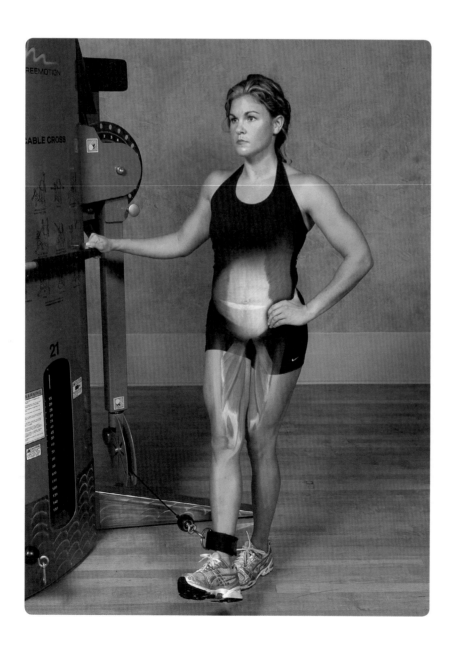

Cable Hip Adduction

Alignment and Positioning

1. Strap one cable to the inside ankle, and stand with the opposite foot straight ahead, aligned directly under the hip, and with the knee slightly bent.

2. Begin with the movement leg about 45 degrees out from the body and the inside hand resting lightly on the bar for balance assistance.

3. Begin with the shoulders back, the spine and head in good posture, and the pelvis level. Draw a deep breath.

Motion and Stabilization

1. Slowly begin to exhale, activate the core, and pull the leg in and slightly across the body while maintaining proper posture and pelvic position.

2. Hold this position, and continue to exhale and to contract the core, trunk, and hip adductors.

3. Slowly begin to inhale, and allow the leg to be pulled back out to the starting position while maintaining proper posture and pelvic positioning.

Trainer Techniques

1. Monitor spine, pelvic, knee, and ankle positioning, hip motion

2. Cue hip adductors (both legs)

3. Spot on lower leg

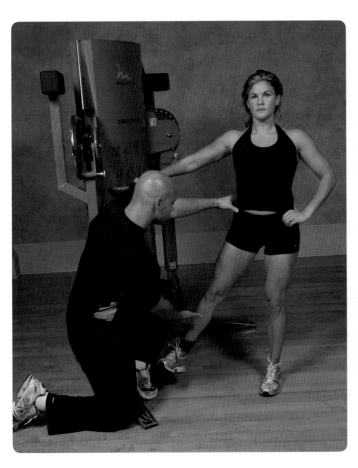

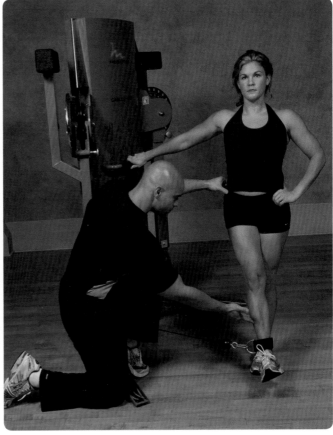

Cable Knee Extension

This exercise loads the extension movement of the knee, targeting the quadriceps. However, the hip flexor of the movement leg, as well as the hip extensors and abductors of the stationary leg, will also be challenged as assistors and stabilizers. Core and trunk muscles will also be challenged to help stabilize the pelvis and spine. More or less stabilization from these muscles is required depending on the amount of arm use. An active stretch of the hamstrings and gastrocnemius of the movement leg can also be accomplished with proper pelvic-spinal positioning and range of motion.

Target Muscles

Knee extensors (quadriceps), hip flexors, anterior oblique subsystem

Joint Motions

Hip flexion, knee extension

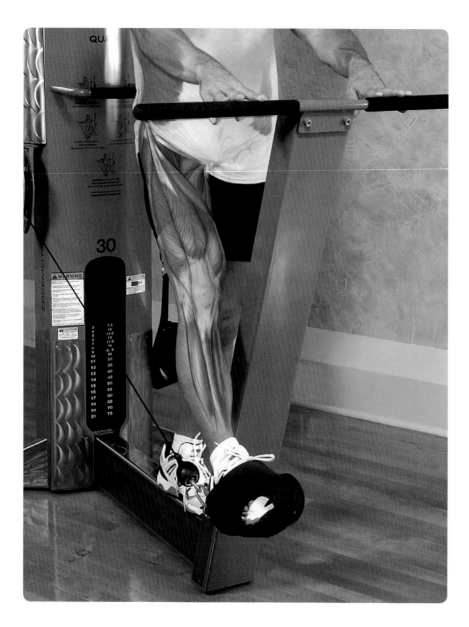

Alignment and Positioning

1. Stand with your weight on one leg and with the toe or ankle of the other leg in the strap, depending on the type of cable machine being used.

2. Begin with the movement leg slightly behind the stationary leg. Position the trunk in good posture.

3. Draw a deep breath, and begin with a slight bend in the hip and knee of the stationary leg.

Motion and Stabilization

1. Begin to exhale, activate the core, flex the hip to begin to pull the leg forward, and flex the ankle to pull the toes up.

2. Continue to pull the leg up, and begin extending the knee while maintaining posture and contracting the core and trunk muscles.

3. Hold, slowly begin to inhale, and allow the knee to bend and the leg to be pulled back to the starting position while maintaining posture.

Trainer Techniques

1. Monitor spine, pelvic, knee, and ankle positioning, knee motion

2. Cue hip flexors, quadriceps

3. Spot on lower leg

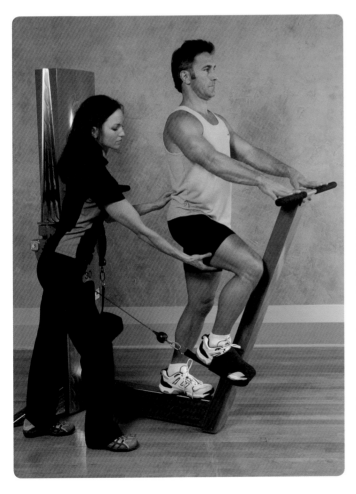 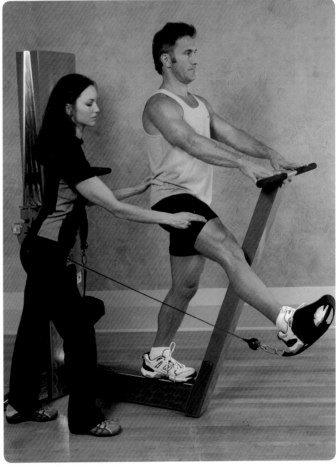

Machine Knee Extension

This exercise isolates knee extension and directly loads the quadriceps muscles. This exercise may be used to accomplish hypertrophy goals, to pre-fatigue the quadriceps, to do rehabilitation work, or to simply add overall volume to a leg program. However, since the knee action is performed in a seated and completely externally stabilized position, the carryover strength and transference of this exercise are limited. Caution should be used when selecting the amount of resistance, because this machine places a direct shearing force across the knee proportional to the load.

Target Muscles

Knee extensors (quadriceps)

Joint Motions

Knee extension

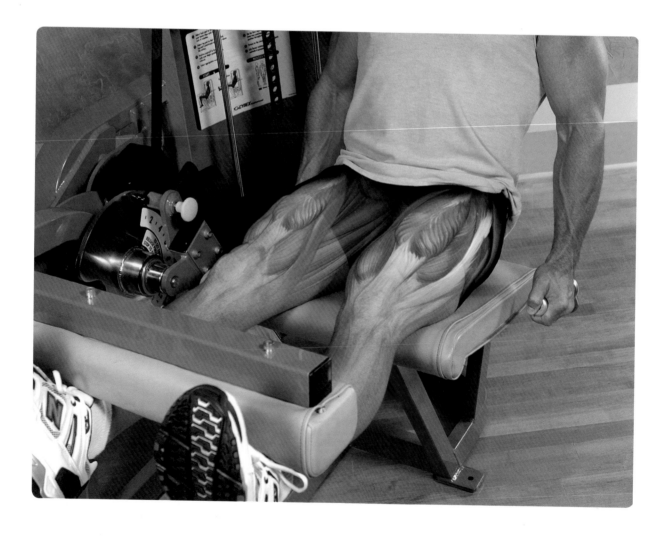

Alignment and Positioning

1. Set the seat so that the knee joint is aligned with the axis and the pad is pressing against the shin.

2. Sit upright or lean against the back pad with good posture so that a full extension of the knee is not quite possible when maintaining the natural arch in the lower back. (Positioning is related to hamstring flexibility.)

3. Begin with the knee flexed no more than 90 degrees and aligned with the toes. Draw a deep breath.

Motion and Stabilization

1. Begin to exhale, activate the core, slightly flex the hips, and then begin to pull the lower legs up and the toes back.

2. Continue to pull the lower legs up and the toes back until the knees are almost locked (while maintaining good upper body posture), which should create a light stretch on the hamstrings.

3. Hold, then slowly inhale and allow the legs to be pushed down to the starting position while maintaining posture.

Trainer Techniques

1. Monitor spine, pelvic, hip, and knee positioning, knee motion

2. Cue quadriceps

3. Spot on pad of machine (assist or resist)

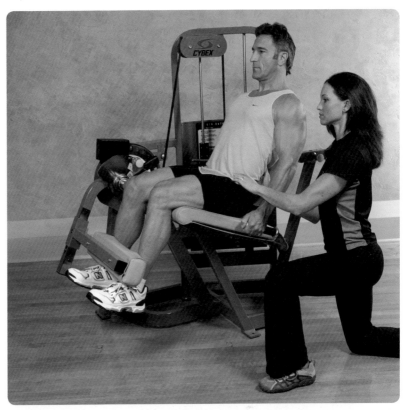

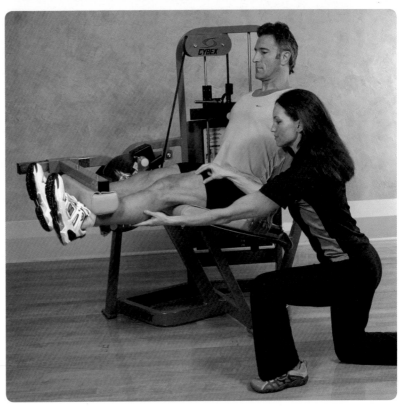

Cable Knee Flexion

This exercise loads hip extension along with knee flexion to better target the hamstrings and hip extensors of the movement leg. The hip flexors and hip abductors of the stationary leg are also challenged as stabilizers. Core and trunk muscles will also be challenged to help stabilize the pelvis and spine, with the amount depending on arm use and hand positioning. An active stretch of the hip flexor muscles of the movement leg can also be accomplished with proper hip positioning and technique.

Target Muscles

Knee flexors (hamstrings), hip extensors, posterior oblique subsystem

Joint Motions

Hip extension, knee flexion

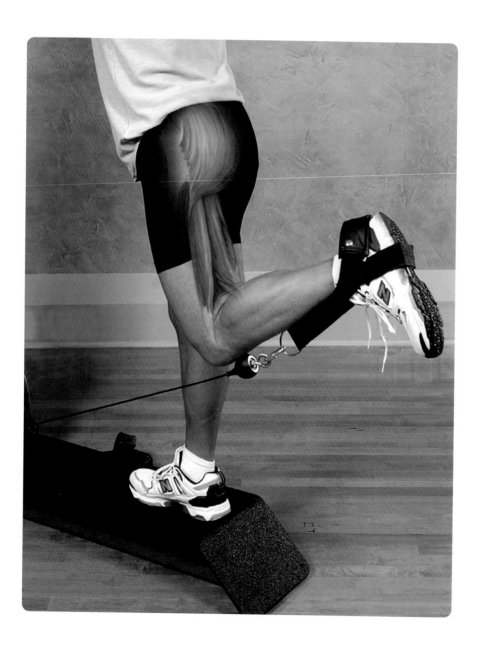

Alignment and Positioning

1. Stand with your weight on one leg and with the foot or ankle of the other leg in the strap, depending on the machine being used.

2. Begin with the movement leg in front of the stationary leg. Position the trunk in good posture.

3. Draw a deep breath, and begin with a slight bend in the knee and hip of the stationary leg.

Motion and Stabilization

1. Begin to exhale, activate the core, begin to extend the hip by pulling the leg back, and stabilize the ankle.

2. Continue to pull the leg back and then flex the knee to about 90 degrees, causing a slight stretch on the hip flexors, while maintaining good posture and further activating the core.

3. Hold, then slowly inhale and allow the leg to be pulled back to the starting position while maintaining posture.

Trainer Techniques

1. Monitor spine, pelvic, knee, and ankle positioning, knee motion

2. Cue hip extensors, hamstrings

3. Spot on lower leg

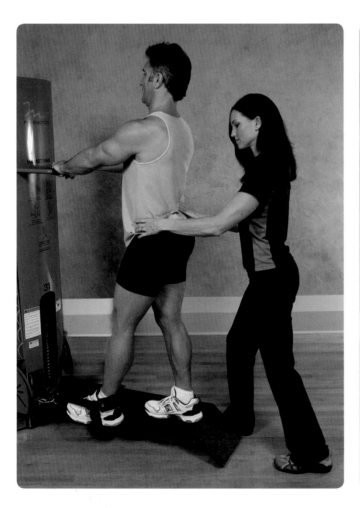
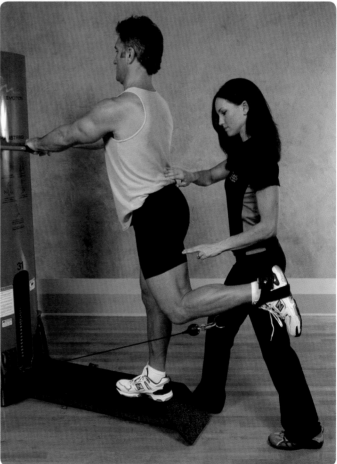

Machine Knee Flexion

This exercise isolates knee flexion and directly targets the hamstring muscles. This exercise may be helpful for achieving hypertrophy goals, working on isolated strengthening of the hamstrings, or simply adding overall volume to a leg program. Knee extension is a resisted movement in squats, presses, and lunges, so a certain amount of isolated knee flexion may be needed to help balance overall strength of the knees. However, isolated joint movements performed in externally stabilized environments have little transference to life uses. Caution should be used when selecting the amount of resistance and prescribing the volume for these types of exercises.

Target Muscles

Knee flexors (hamstrings)

Joint Motions

Knee flexion

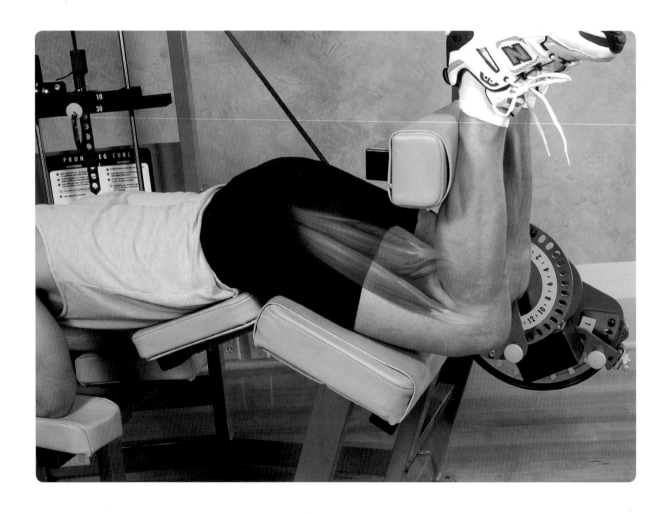

Alignment and Positioning

1. Lie prone on a bench so that the knee joint is aligned with the axis and the pad is positioned below the gastrocnemius and above the Achilles tendon.

2. Position the trunk and neck in proper posture, with the head off the pad looking straight down and with the chin tucked.

3. Begin with the knees slightly bent, the pelvis pressed against the pad, and the feet straight and stabilized. Draw a deep breath.

Motion and Stabilization

1. Begin to exhale, activate the core, press the pelvis tight into the pad (slightly raising the knees off the pad), and begin to pull the lower legs up.

2. Continue to slightly lift the knees, and pull the lower legs up so that the knee is flexed about 90 degrees while maintaining posture and further contracting the core and trunk muscles.

3. Hold, then slowly inhale and allow the legs to be pulled down to the starting position while maintaining pelvic-spinal positioning.

Trainer Techniques

1. Monitor spine, pelvic, hip, and knee positioning, knee motion

2. Cue hamstrings

3. Spot on pad of machine (assist or resist)

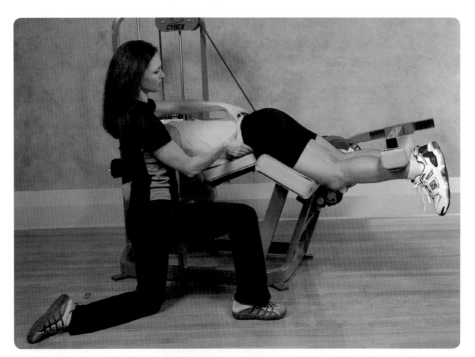

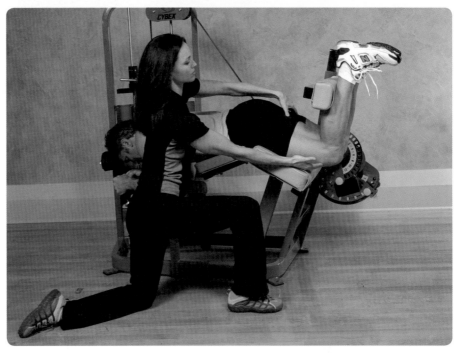

Dumbbell One-Leg Ankle Extension

This exercise is an often overlooked option for training the ankle extensors and is more transferable to life demands than machine calf extension movements. The amount of balance challenge can be moderated by using a hand to assist. Options for strengthening ankle eversion or inversion are also available with this exercise through voluntary ankle control that is not possible when using most machines.

Target Muscles

Ankle extensors (triceps surae)

Joint Motions

Ankle extension (plantar flexion)

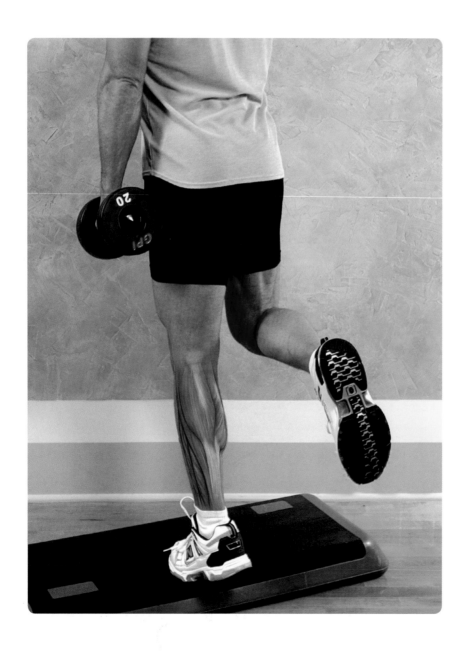

Dumbbell One-Leg Ankle Extension

Alignment and Positioning

1. Stand in good posture with the ball of one foot securely positioned on a step, with the toes and entire leg pointed straight ahead. The other leg should be slightly bent.

2. Hold a dumbbell in the opposite or same-side arm depending on the degree of balance challenge desired. Place the opposite hand lightly on a wall or stable object for slight balance assistance.

3. Begin with a slight bend in the knee, the ankle flexed, and the heel just below the ball of the foot. Then inhale.

Motion and Stabilization

1. Begin to exhale, activate the core, and extend the ankle to lift the body up, keeping the ankle from rolling out and the weight over the ball of the foot.

2. Extend the ankle as far as possible, keeping it stable and lifting the body while maintaining good posture and further contracting the core and trunk muscles.

3. Hold, then slowly inhale and allow the body to lower down to the starting position while maintaining proper posture and ankle positioning.

Trainer Techniques

1. Monitor spine, pelvic, knee, and ankle positioning, ankle motion

2. Cue gastrocs

3. Spot under heel or possibly under rib cage

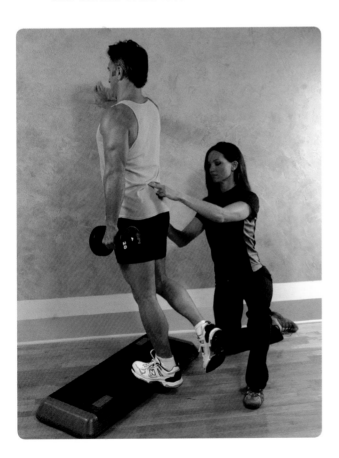
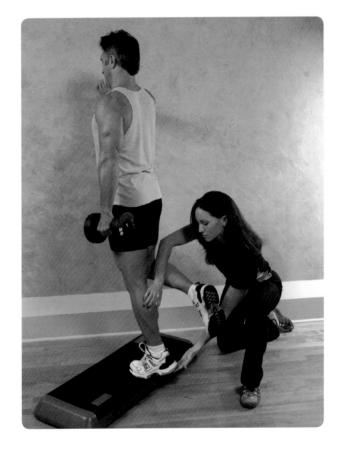

Machine Straight-Leg Ankle Extension

This exercise can be used to isolate ankle extension and better load the calves. This exercise may be helpful for achieving hypertrophy goals, working on specific ankle strengthening, or if using this particular machine, concurrently strengthening ankle inversion or eversion along with ankle extension. Though beneficial for certain aesthetic- or performance-based goals, isolated machine training exercises may not transfer much to meeting the demands placed on the ankle during life situations or during higher speed dynamic movements. This exercise can also be done with one leg at a time for isolateral strengthening of the ankles.

Target Muscles

Ankle extensors (triceps surae)

Joint Motions

Ankle extension (plantar flexion)

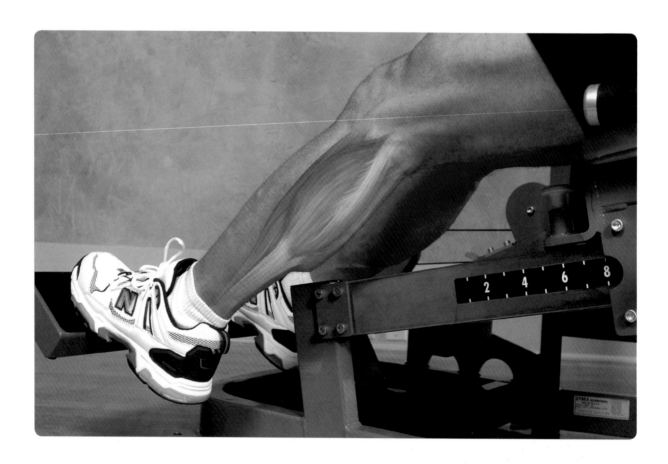

Machine Straight-Leg Ankle Extension

Alignment and Positioning

1. Sit with the balls of the feet securely positioned on the foot pedals, with the toes and legs aligned straight.

2. Pull the shoulders back, position the spine in good posture, and draw a deep breath.

3. Begin with a slight bend in the knees, and flex the ankles so that the heels are slightly in front of the balls of the feet.

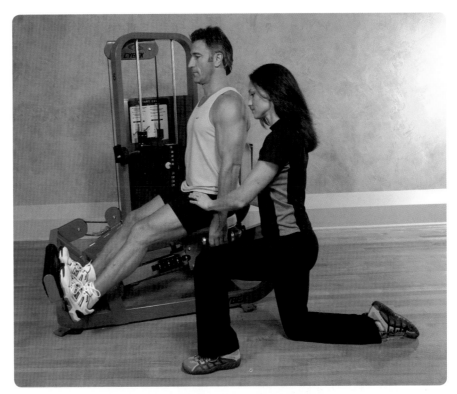

Motion and Stabilization

1. Begin to exhale, activate the core, and extend the ankles to press the foot pedals out while maintaining pelvic-spinal positioning.

2. Press the pedals out as far as possible while keeping the ankles from rolling in or out. Keep the pressure through the balls of the feet, and further contract the core and trunk muscles.

3. Hold, then slowly inhale and allow the ankles to flex and the pedals to return to the starting position while maintaining good posture.

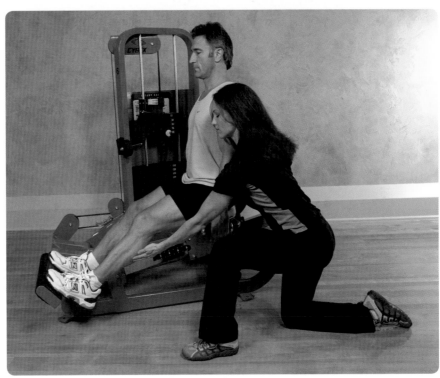

Trainer Techniques

1. Monitor lumbar spine, pelvic, knee, and ankle positioning, ankle motion

2. Cue gastrocs

3. Spot on foot plate of machine (assist or resist)

Machine Bent-Leg Ankle Extension

This exercise targets strengthening of the ankle extensors, with emphasis placed primarily on the soleus. Because the gastrocnemius muscles are two-joint muscles, when bending the knee they are preshortened and become active insufficient, leaving the soleus to carry most of the load. With any calf exercise, you should make sure to avoid having the weight force the athlete's ankles to flex more than they could actively flex on their own power. This exercise may be helpful for achieving certain aesthetic-based or performance-based goals, but it will transfer little to the life demands regularly placed on the ankles.

Target Muscles

Ankle extensors (triceps surae)

Joint Motions

Ankle extension (plantar flexion)

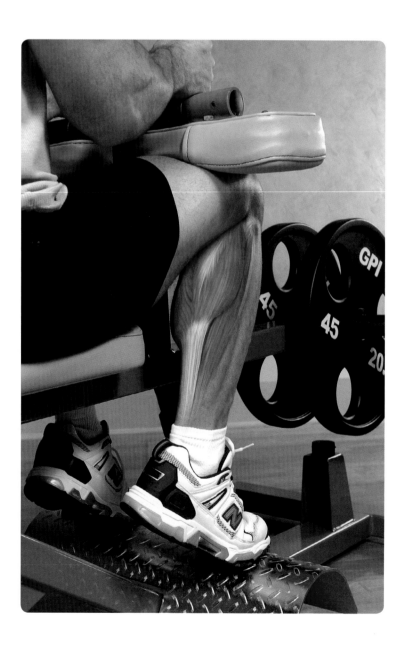

Machine Bent-Leg Ankle Extension

Alignment and Positioning

1. Sit with the balls of the feet securely positioned on the step, with the toes and legs aligned straight ahead.

2. Place the knees under the pads, pull the shoulders back, and position the spine in good posture.

3. Begin with the heels slightly below the balls of the feet. Draw a deep breath.

Motion and Stabilization

1. Begin to exhale, activate the core, and extend the ankles to lift the knees and the weight.

2. Press up as far as possible, keeping the ankles from rolling out and keeping the weight over the balls of the feet. Continue to contract the core and trunk muscles.

3. Hold, then slowly inhale and allow the legs to lower down to the starting position while maintaining proper posture and ankle positioning.

Trainer Techniques

1. Monitor lumbar spine, pelvic, knee, and ankle positioning, ankle motion

2. Cue soleus

3. Spot on resistance lever of machine (assist or resist)

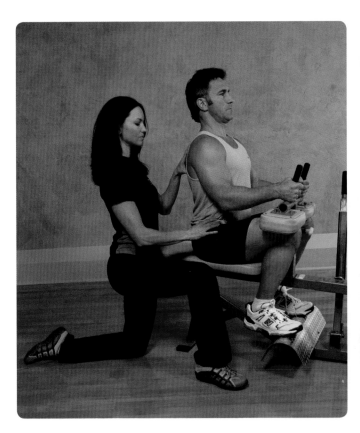
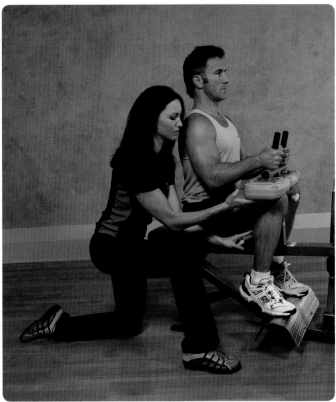

Machine Ankle Flexion

This exercise isolates strengthening of the ankle flexors, emphasizing the tibialis anterior. Strengthening exercises are often performed for the ankle extensors in training programs, but these important flexors of the ankle are often overlooked. Maintaining a relative strength balance around any joint is a key for optimal performance of the joint and for decreasing the risk of potential injury. This exercise may also serve as an active-stretching exercise of the gastrocnemius and Achilles tendon when done properly and with a full concentric range of motion.

Target Muscles

Ankle flexors (tibialis anterior), flexor digitorums, flexor hallucis

Joint Motions

Ankle flexion (dorsiflexion)

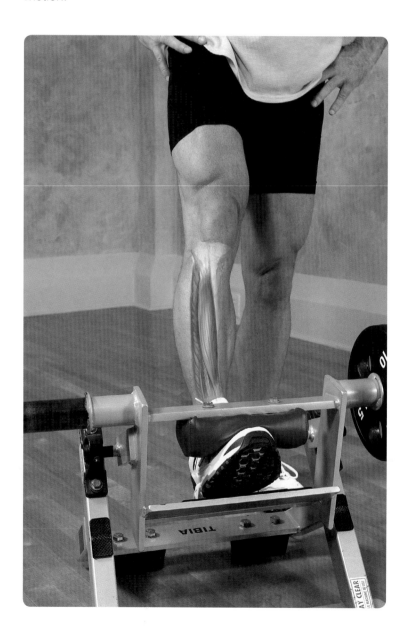

Alignment and Positioning

1. Stand with the foot placed securely under the pad, with the ankle aligned with the axis of the machine.

2. Straighten and lock the knee of the working leg, and position the foot parallel to the ground.

3. Stand in good posture while balancing on one leg. Draw a deep breath.

Motion and Stabilization

1. Begin to exhale, activate the core, and flex the ankle to pull the foot up and back.

2. Flex the ankle as far as possible while keeping the toes relaxed and the knee locked. Further contract the core and trunk muscles.

3. Hold, then slowly inhale and allow the foot to lower down to the starting position while maintaining proper posture and ankle positioning.

Trainer Techniques

1. Monitor pelvic, knee, and ankle positioning, ankle motion

2. Cue tibialis anterior

3. Spot on resistance lever of machine (assist or resist)

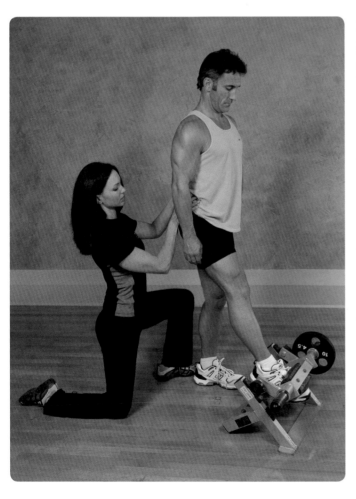
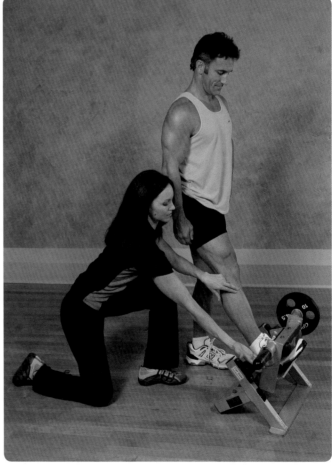

Upper-Body Pushing Exercises

In this chapter, several exercises are presented that target and strengthen the scapular, shoulder, elbow, and wrist muscles that are responsible for providing pushing forces. Integration of core and trunk muscle stabilization is an essential element of technique for many of these exercises. Pushing exercises are classified as general movement patterns, but some specific movement patterns that are used for isolating the triceps (which assist in pushing movements) are also included in this chapter. Upper body structure and function, along with specific muscle physiology and all biomechanical factors, were considered when developing the instructions for all elements of technique, such as alignment, positioning, motion, stabilization, and suggested breathing method.

These exercise selections vary in their difficulty of stabilization or movement demands in order to provide a well-balanced collection of movements to challenge individuals of all strength and fitness levels. Some exercises are more suited for addressing performance-based goals while others are ideal for achieving more aesthetic-based goals. Variations and modifications that will increase or decrease the level of challenge are also provided in the description section for many exercises. Consider the steps below when selecting exercises as they were derived through combining information relative to exercise technique presented in chapter 4 along with the exercise selection process presented in chapter 5 in order to help select and instruct the efficient performance of each exercise.

1. Identify the goal (aesthetic- or performance-based)
2. Select the desired movement pattern (general movement pattern or specific movement pattern)
3. Select the muscle groups to be targeted (muscle synergies or isolated muscles)
4. Identify alignment of the forces (pull of the muscles vs. pull or push of the resistance)
5. Consider the positioning options (proprioception vs. neural availability)
6. Focus on stabilization (more important than the actual movement)
7. Use and control the planned tempo (affects type of strength, is a component of volume)
8. Integrate breathing method or control

Dumbbell Horizontal Press

This exercise is a horizontal plane press that targets the chest and anterior shoulder muscles. Dumbbells provide for more freedom of movement, require more demand from scapular and shoulder stabilizers, and reduce some of the additional shearing and compressive forces associated with barbell and machine presses. Dumbbells also allow more user options for accomplishing different goals, such as unilateral movements, alternate movements, piston movements, or using different loads in each hand. This exercise is presented with a retracted scapular positioning to decrease stress on the shoulder joint, because natural scapular movement and rhythm are not possible while on a bench.

Target Muscles

Sternal pectoralis major, clavicular pectoralis major, anterior deltoid, triceps

Joint Motions

Shoulder horizontal flexion, elbow extension

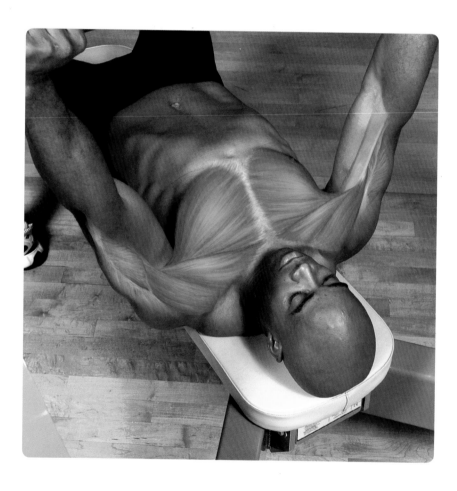

Alignment and Positioning

1. Lie supine on a bench, with good posture, a natural arch in the lower spine, and the feet braced firmly on the floor or on a step.

2. Retract the shoulder blades slightly together, and position the dumbbells horizontal to the body and aligned over the shoulders.

3. Begin with the elbows pointed outward, the wrists straight, and the core and trunk muscles contracted.

Motion and Stabilization

1. Begin to inhale. Slowly lower the arms and allow the hands to separate, keeping them just inside the elbows, while maintaining pelvic-spinal positioning.

2. Continue to lower the arms until the upper arm is about parallel with the floor, with the hands slightly inside the elbows.

3. Hold, slowly exhale, activate the core, and press the arms and dumbbells back to the starting position while maintaining proper posture and scapular positioning.

Trainer Techniques

1. Monitor spine and scapular positioning, shoulder and elbow motion

2. Cue pectoralis

3. Spot under the elbows or on wrists

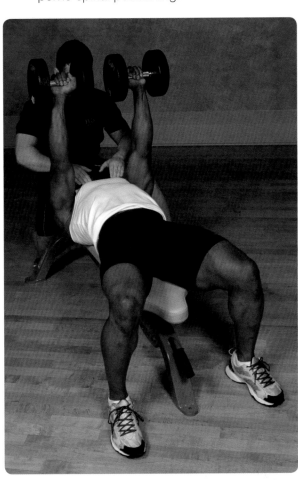 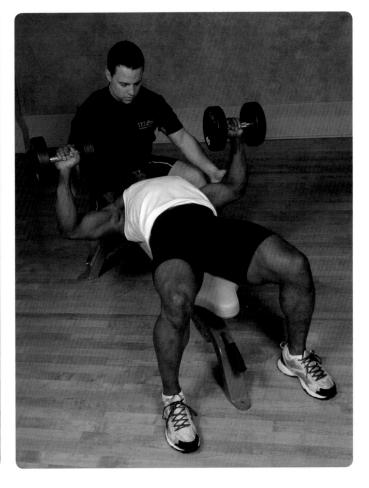

Barbell Horizontal Press

This exercise is conducted primarily in the horizontal plane and targets the chest, shoulder, and triceps muscles. Pressing with a barbell forces a closed-chain action of the arms that may enable the lifter to move heavier loads than with dumbbells but also inherently adds shearing and compressive forces that can stress and increase wear on the shoulder and elbow joints. These forces can be further complicated when using poor alignment with hand positioning, increasing the range of motion, using too fast of tempo, and lifting heavier loads, so be sure to monitor these as the athlete performs this exercise. Technique, goal determination, and risk-to-benefit assessment should be carefully considered when selecting this exercise and when increasing load or volume.

Target Muscles

Sternal pectoralis major, clavicular pectoralis major, anterior deltoid, triceps

Joint Motions

Shoulder horizontal flexion, elbow extension

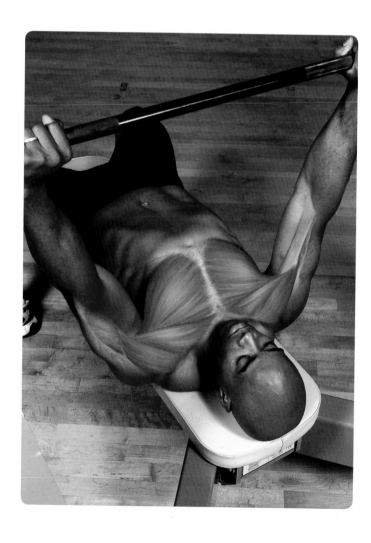

Alignment and Positioning

1. Lie supine on a bench, with good posture and with the feet braced firmly on the floor or on a step.

2. Retract the shoulder blades slightly together, and place the hands on the bar at a width that will create a 90-degree angle at the elbow when the upper arm is parallel to the floor.

3. Begin with the bar over the chest, the elbows pointed out, the wrists straight, and the core and trunk muscles contracted.

Motion and Stabilization

1. Begin to inhale. Slowly lower the arms and the bar while keeping the elbows under the bar and maintaining pelvic-spinal positioning.

2. Continue to lower the bar down until the upper arm is about parallel with the floor, with the hands just inside the elbows.

3. Hold, slowly begin to exhale, activate the core, and press the arms and the barbell back to the starting position while maintaining proper posture and scapular positioning.

Trainer Techniques

1. Monitor spine and scapular positioning, shoulder and elbow motion

2. Cue pectoralis

3. Spot under the elbows or on the bar

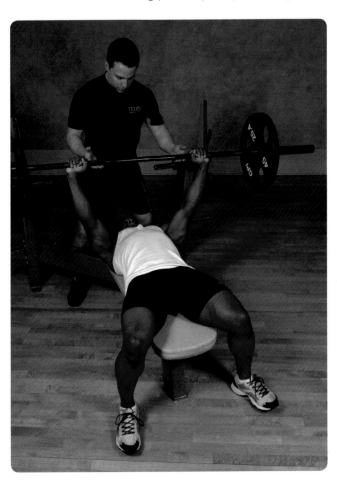

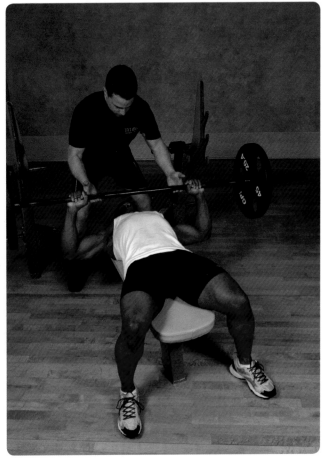

Dumbbell Swiss Ball One-Arm Horizontal Press

This exercise targets the upper chest and anterior shoulder muscles. Working on a Swiss ball together with unequally loading the body places an additional demand on the core, trunk rotators, and associated hip muscles to maintain proper posture against the applied rotational force. Exercises done on the ball also require more neck flexor strength because the head will be unsupported throughout the exercise. This exercise can be done at different body and shoulder angles for more or less chest emphasis. It can also be performed with two arms, alternate movements, piston movements, or with a different amount of weight in each hand for varied training effects.

Target Muscles

Sternal pectoralis major, clavicular pectoralis major, anterior deltoid, triceps

Joint Motions

Shoulder horizontal flexion (inclined angle), elbow extension

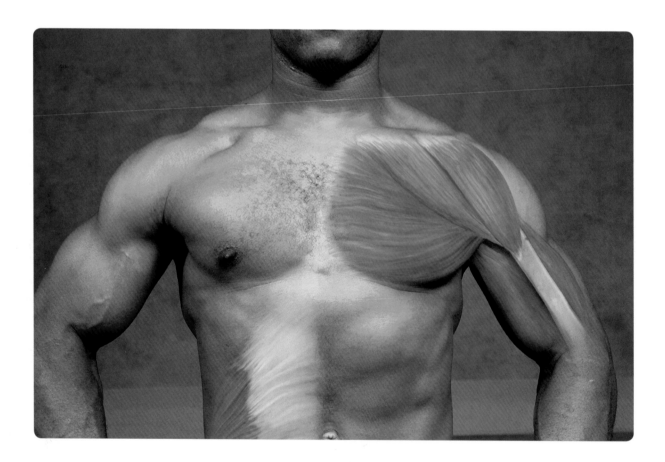

Dumbbell Swiss Ball One-Arm Horizontal Press

Alignment and Positioning

1. Position the body at a 45-degree angle on a Swiss ball, with good posture and with the feet braced firmly on the floor or on a step.
2. Pull the shoulders slightly together, and position the dumbbell horizontal to the body and aligned straight over the shoulder.
3. Begin with the elbow pointed out, the wrist straight, and the core and trunk muscles contracted.

Motion and Stabilization

1. Begin to inhale, and lower the arm while keeping the hand slightly inside the elbow and avoiding any rotation of the trunk.

2. Continue to lower the arm until the upper arm is about parallel with the floor, with the hand slightly inside the elbow. Maintain good posture.
3. Hold, slowly exhale, activate the core, and press the arm and dumbbell back to the starting position while maintaining proper posture.

Trainer Techniques

1. Monitor spine, pelvic, and scapular positioning, shoulder and elbow motion
2. Cue upper pectoralis
3. Spot under the elbow or on the wrist

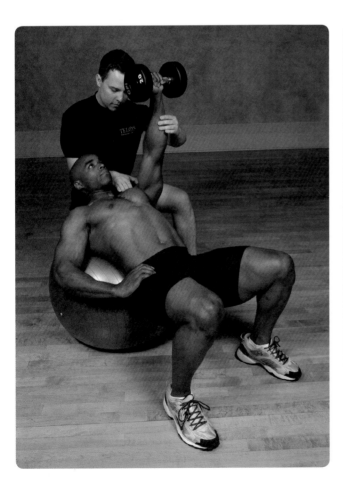
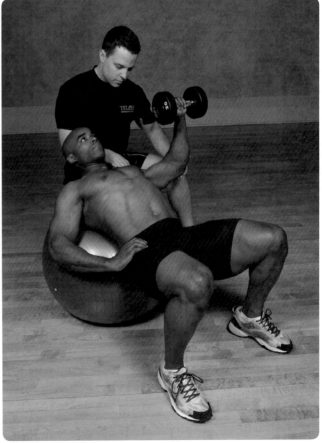

Cable One-Arm Decline Horizontal Press

This exercise targets the lower chest and anterior shoulder muscles. Pressing with one arm while in the lunge position also targets the same-side obliques, associated core and abdominal muscles, and the contralateral hip adductors and flexors, which can collectively be considered the anterior oblique subsystem (AOS). This exercise may not be a high contributor for achieving certain aesthetic goals, such as chest hypertrophy, but it is valuable for addressing performance-related goals such as improved pelvic-spinal stabilization or preparation for powerful rotational movements. This should be a prerequisite for the Cable Trunk Rotation With Press exercise presented in chapter 7.

Target Muscles

Sternal pectoralis major, clavicular pectoralis major, anterior deltoid, triceps, anterior oblique subsystem

Joint Motions

Shoulder horizontal flexion (decline angle), elbow extension

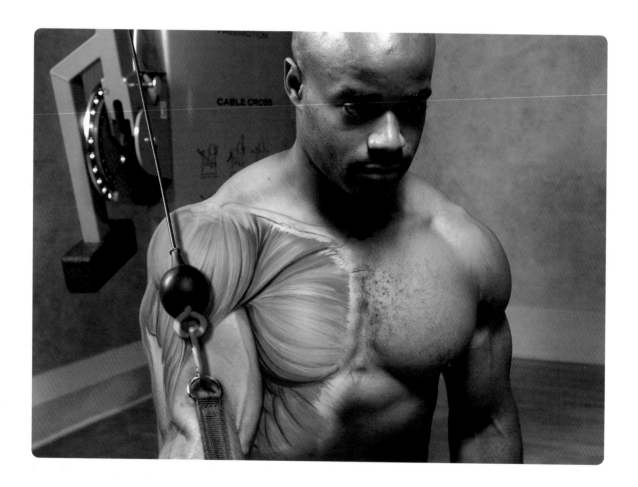

Cable One-Arm Decline Horizontal Press

Alignment and Positioning

1. Stand in a lunge position, with the feet about shoulder-width apart and the trunk leaned forward in good posture.

2. Position the cable handle down, perpendicular to the body, and aligned straight with the shoulder and pulley.

3. Begin with the elbow straight and pointed out, the wrist straight, and the core and trunk muscles contracted.

Motion and Stabilization

1. Begin to inhale, and slowly allow the arm to be pulled out and up while keeping the hand slightly inside the elbow and avoiding any movement of the trunk.

2. Continue to have the arm pulled back until the elbow is about even with the shoulder, with the hand slightly inside the elbow.

3. Hold, slowly exhale, activate the core, and press the arm back down and in to the starting position while maintaining proper posture.

Trainer Techniques

1. Monitor spine and pelvic positioning, scapular, shoulder, and elbow motion

2. Cue pectoralis

3. Spot on the wrist or under rib cage

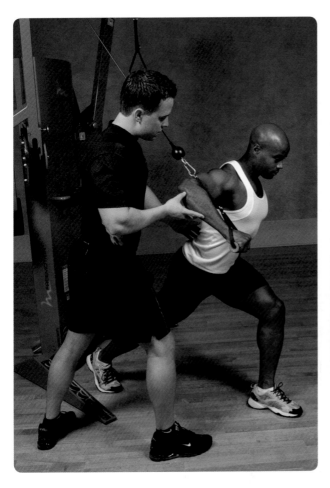 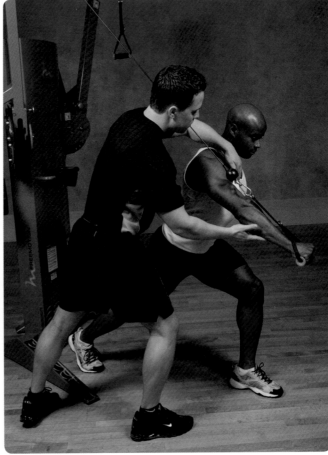

Squat Rack Decline Push-Up

This exercise also targets the chest, shoulder, and triceps muscles. Performing push-ups forces the same closed-chain action that occurs with a barbell press and can be stressful to the shoulder joints; this can be compounded with certain hand positioning and alignment options so be sure the athlete has been properly instructed. The push-up position also places a load on the abdominal and hip flexors for stabilization requirements. Challenge can be decreased or increased by raising or lowering the angle of the body before beginning. Performing a push-up with one foot off the ground increases the balance challenge and increases the load on the hip flexor of the stationary leg.

Target Muscles

Sternal pectoralis major; clavicular pectoralis major; anterior deltoid; triceps; core, trunk, and hip flexors

Joint Motions

Shoulder horizontal flexion, elbow extension

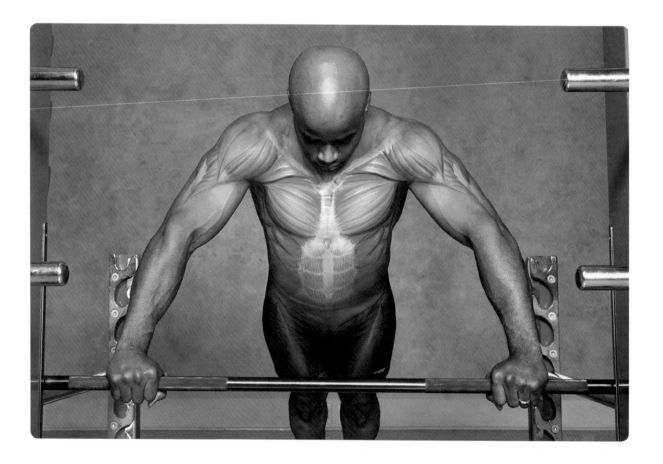

Alignment and Positioning

1. Position the bar at the desired height for the appropriate resistance. Place the hands at a width that will form a 90-degree angle at the elbow when the upper arm is parallel to the floor.

2. Align the body at a perpendicular angle to the arms, with the balls of the feet firmly pressed against the floor.

3. Begin with good posture, the elbows pointed out, the wrists straight, and the core and trunk muscles contracted.

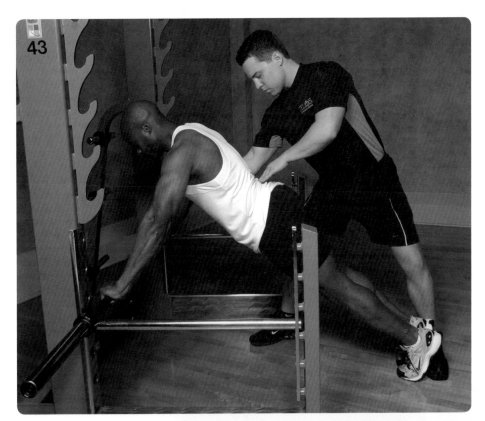

Motion and Stabilization

1. Begin to inhale, and allow the body to lower while keeping the elbows pointed out and the spine and pelvis stabilized.

2. Continue to lower the body down until an approximate 90-degree angle is formed at the elbow.

3. Hold, slowly exhale, activate the core, and press the body back up to the starting position while maintaining proper posture.

Trainer Techniques

1. Monitor spine and pelvic positioning, scapular, shoulder, and elbow motion

2. Cue pectoralis

3. Spot under pelvic girdle or under rib cage

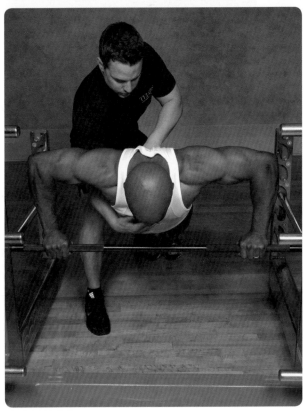

Dumbbell Incline Median Press

This exercise targets the anterior deltoids but also works some upper chest muscles and the triceps. The median plane is the most common plane a person moves in throughout the day. However, pushing exercises in the median plane are often neglected in resistance training programs. This exercise can be performed at a variety of body angles depending on the lifter's active range of motion abilities. This exercise is presented with a stabilized scapular position because natural scapular movement and rhythm are not possible when braced against a bench. The exercise can also be performed with a single arm, alternate movements, piston movements, and offset loads for varied training effects.

Target Muscles

Anterior deltoids, clavicular pectoralis major, triceps

Joint Motions

Shoulder flexion, elbow extension

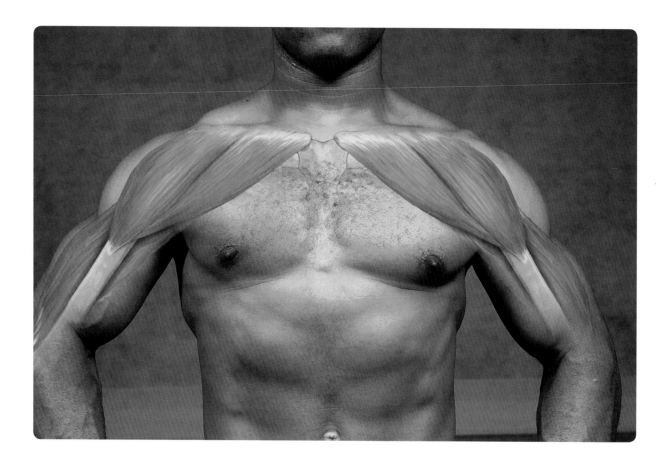

Dumbbell Incline Median Press

Alignment and Positioning

1. Position the body with good posture on a bench at a 30- to 80-degree angle depending on shoulder mobility and desired goals.

2. Begin with the dumbbells parallel to the body and just over the elbows, which are also aligned parallel to the body.

3. Slightly retract and depress the shoulder blades, lift the chest, and create a natural arch in the lower back. Draw a deep breath.

Motion and Stabilization

1. Begin to exhale, activate the core, and slowly press the arms up, keeping the dumbbells and the elbows aligned parallel with the body.

2. Continue to press the arms up until directly over the shoulders while maintaining pelvic-spinal and scapular positioning.

3. Hold, then slowly begin to inhale, and lower the arms back to the starting position while maintaining proper posture.

Trainer Techniques

1. Monitor spine and pelvic positioning, scapular, shoulder, and elbow motion

2. Cue anterior deltoids and upper pectoralis

3. Spot under elbows or on wrists

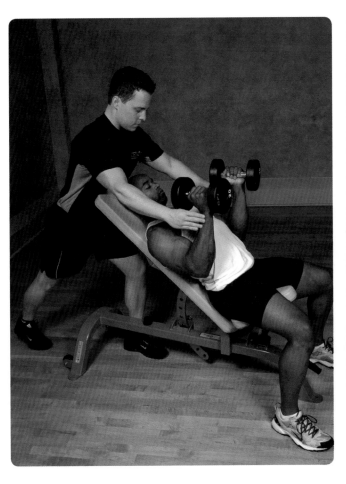
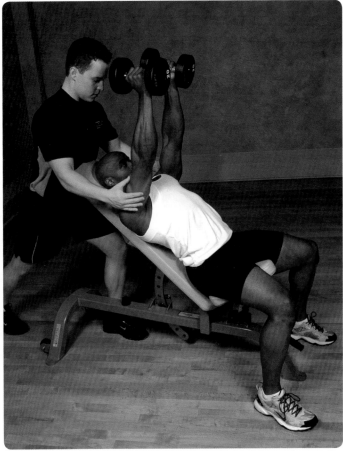

Dumbbell Frontal Press

This exercise targets the anterior shoulder, the triceps, and, to a lesser extent, the upper chest. However, frontal plane pressing requires specific scapular-thoracic and scapular-humeral rhythm that subsequently integrates serratus anterior, levator scapula, and trapezius muscles as well. The trunk is not braced against a bench for this exercise in order to allow for proper scapular motion. Therefore it requires increased core, trunk, and hip musculature to meet balance and stabilization demands. This exercise can be performed with alternate movements, piston movements, offset loads, or with one arm for varied goals.

Target Muscles

Anterior deltoids, clavicular pectoralis major, triceps, trapezius, other scapular upward rotators

Joint Motions

Shoulder frontal flexion (abduction), elbow extension

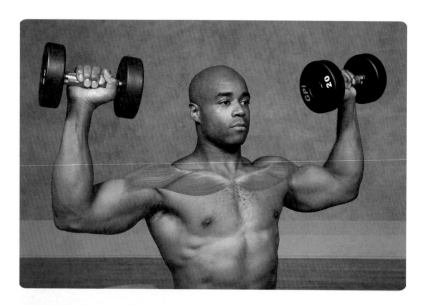

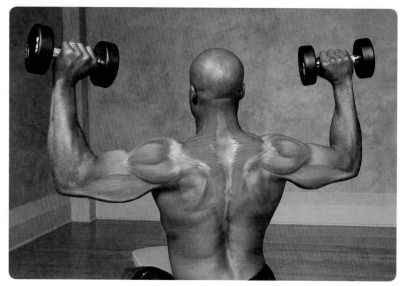

Dumbbell Frontal Press

Alignment and Positioning

1. Sit in good posture with the hips and knees flexed about 90 degrees and a natural arch in the lower back.

2. Bring the arms up and out to the sides of the body, with the upper arms about parallel to the floor, the elbows flexed about 90 degrees, and with the dumbbells level and just inside the elbows.

3. Slightly lift the chest, stabilize posture, and inhale.

Motion and Stabilization

1. Begin to exhale, activate the core, and slowly press the arms up, keeping the dumbbells and the elbows aligned with the body.

2. Continue to press the arms up and over until directly over the shoulders. Attempt to elevate the shoulder blades as they rotate upward while maintaining pelvic-spinal positioning.

3. Hold, then slowly begin to inhale, and lower the arms back to the starting position while maintaining proper posture.

Trainer Techniques

1. Monitor spine and pelvic positioning, scapular, shoulder, and elbow motion

2. Cue anterior deltoids and upper pectoralis

3. Spot under elbows or on wrists

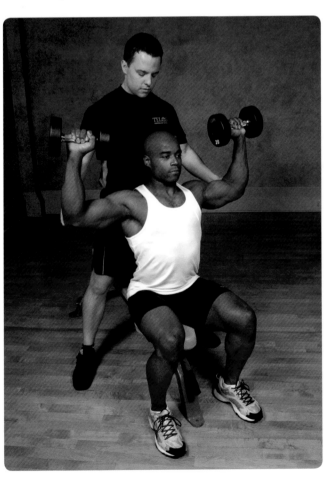
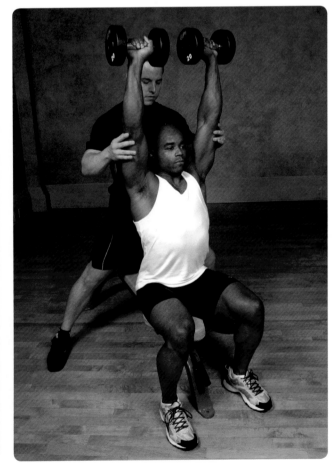

Dumbbell One-Arm and One-Leg Frontal Press

This exercise targets the anterior shoulder, the triceps, and, to a lesser extent, the upper chest. However, frontal plane pressing requires specific scapular-thoracic and scapular-humeral rhythm that subsequently integrates trapezius and other scapular muscles as well. The single-leg positioning demands high levels of involvement for the core, trunk, and hip muscles to stabilize the body, particularly those muscles that make up the lateral subsystem (LS). This exercise can also be performed using the opposite arm, both arms, offset loads, or alternate and piston movements for varied training effects.

Target Muscles

Anterior deltoids, clavicular pectoralis major, triceps, trapezius, other scapular upward rotators, lateral subsystem (hip abductors, contralateral trunk lateral flexors)

Joint Motions

Shoulder frontal flexion (abduction), elbow extension

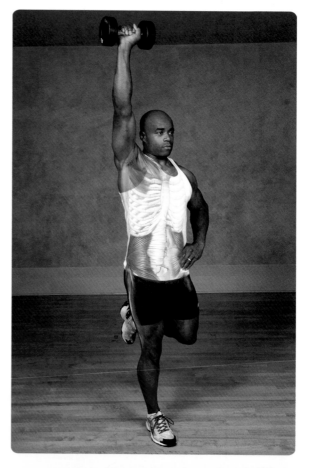

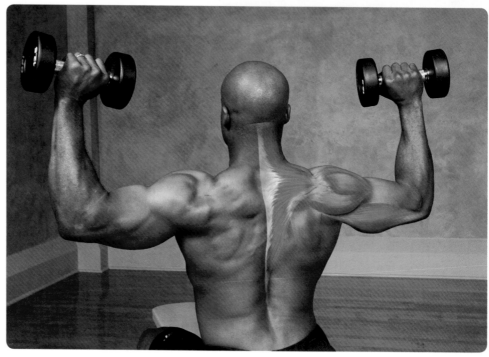

Dumbbell One-Arm and One-Leg Frontal Press

Alignment and Positioning

1. Stand on one leg, with the other foot off the ground. Position the pelvis level and the trunk in good posture.

2. Bring the arm up and out to the side of the body, with the upper arm about parallel to the floor, the elbow flexed about 90 degrees, and the dumbbell level and just inside the elbow.

3. Slightly lift the chest, stabilize posture, and inhale.

Motion and Stabilization

1. Begin to exhale, activate the core, and slowly press the arm up, keeping the dumbbell and the elbow aligned with the body.

2. Continue to press the arm up and over until directly over the shoulder. Attempt to elevate the shoulder blade as it rotates upward while maintaining pelvic-spinal positioning.

3. Hold, then slowly begin to inhale and lower the arm back to the starting position while maintaining proper posture.

Trainer Techniques

1. Monitor spine and pelvic positioning, scapular, shoulder, and elbow motion

2. Cue anterior deltoids and upper pectoralis

3. Spot under elbow or under rib cage

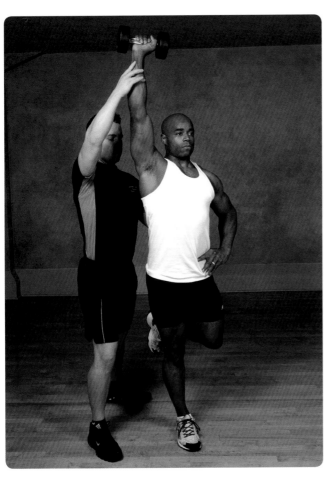
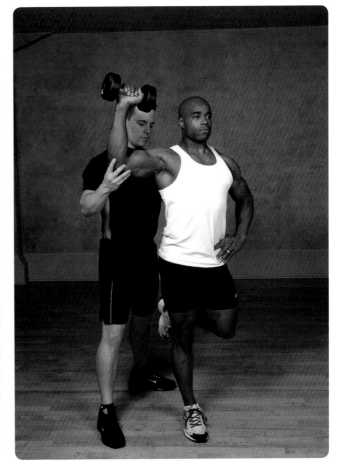

Cable One-Arm 90-Degree Elbow Extension

This exercise targets the triceps muscle group. The flexed shoulder position helps to emphasize the long head of the triceps, and the neutral elbow positioning will target wrist adductors. Performing this exercise in a standing, unbraced position also places a stabilization demand on the core, trunk, and hip muscles. Although isolated elbow extension is most often associated with aesthetic goals, the specific shoulder, elbow, and wrist positioning and the trunk stabilization challenges may help to concurrently progress certain performance goals as well. Two-arm, alternate, and piston movements may be possible options if using certain brands of pulley and cable machines with dual handles.

Target Muscles

Triceps, wrist adductors, shoulder and scapular stabilizers

Joint Motions

Elbow extension

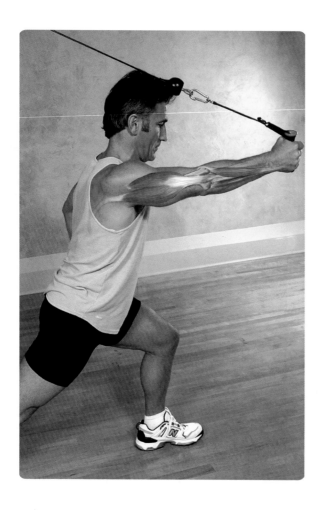

Cable One-Arm 90-Degree Elbow Extension

Alignment and Positioning

1. Hold the handle of the upper cable lengthwise in the hand, and step out into a lunge position.

2. Lean the trunk over to approximately a 45-degree angle, and position the elbow and shoulder at about 90-degree angles, with the lower arm and hand in a neutral position.

3. Begin with the entire spine and neck in good posture. Draw a deep breath.

Motion and Stabilization

1. Begin to exhale, activate the core, and contract the triceps to begin extending the elbow.

2. Continue to fully extend the elbow, keeping the shoulder, scapula, and wrist stabilized and keeping the elbow pointed to the floor.

3. Hold, then slowly inhale and allow the lower arm to be pulled back to the starting position, keeping the shoulder, scapula, and wrist stabilized and the trunk in good posture.

Trainer Techniques

1. Monitor spine, pelvic, and scapular positioning, elbow motion

2. Cue triceps

3. Spot on wrist and upper arm

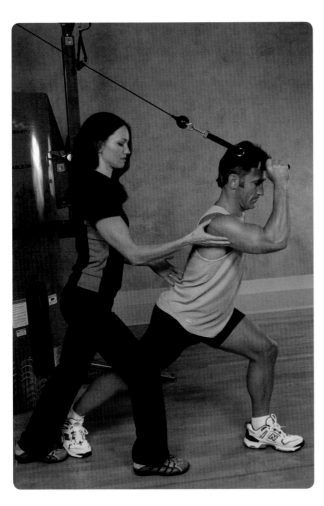 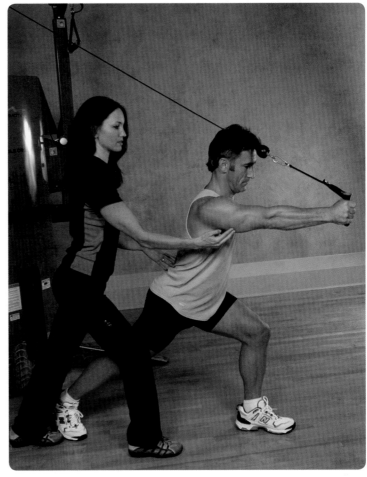

Cable Zero-Degree Elbow Extension

This exercise emphasizes the lateral head of the triceps by using a shoulder position that preshortens the long head of the triceps, making it somewhat active insufficient toward the end of the range of motion. This exercise is often selected primarily for aesthetic-based goals. However, it does require a significant level of stabilization to maintain the recommended scapular depression, scapular retraction, and spinal positioning that will improve postural ability as well as develop the triceps. Note that a curved bar can be used to position the lower arms in a semineutral position that makes it easier to stabilize proper shoulder positioning, which assists with posture and decreases elbow stress.

Target Muscles

Triceps, shoulder and scapular stabilizers

Joint Motions

Elbow extension

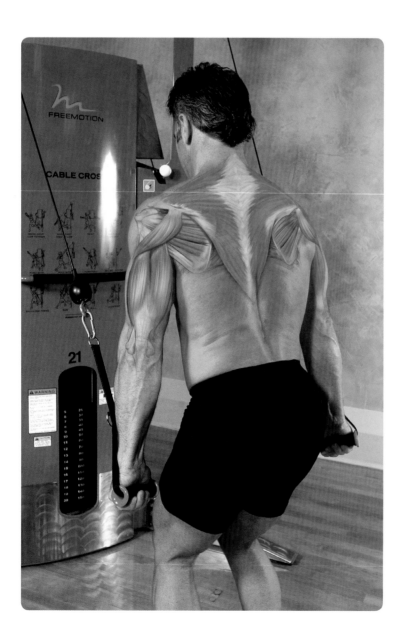

Cable Zero-Degree Elbow Extension

Alignment and Positioning

1. Face the cable column, and grasp the handles with the hands about shoulder-width apart and in a semineutral position.

2. Lean the trunk forward in good posture, flexing at the hips as needed to be aligned parallel with the cable.

3. Pull the elbows to the sides so they are parallel to the body, pointed down, and flexed about 120 degrees. Stabilize the shoulders and inhale.

Motion and Stabilization

1. Begin to exhale, activate the core, and contract the triceps to begin extending the elbows.

2. Continue to fully extend the elbows, keeping the shoulders, scapula, and wrists stabilized and keeping the elbows pointed back.

3. Hold, then slowly inhale and allow the lower arms to be pulled back to the starting position, keeping the shoulders, scapula, and wrists stabilized and the trunk in good posture.

Trainer Techniques

1. Monitor spine, pelvic, and scapular positioning, elbow motion

2. Cue triceps

3. Spot on forearms or upper arms

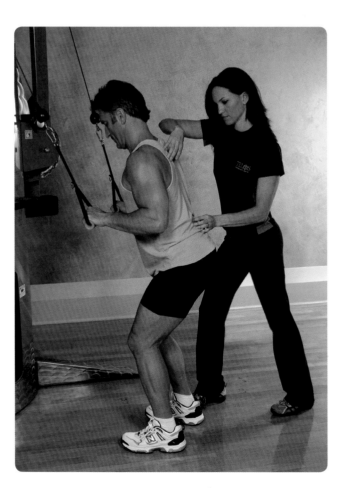
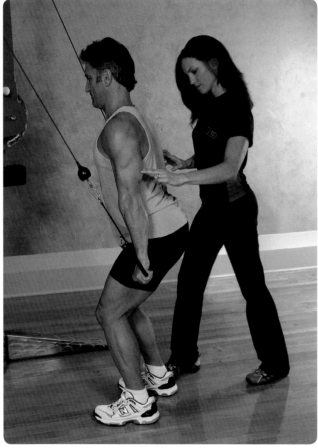

Upper-Body Pulling Exercises

In this chapter, several exercises are presented that target and strengthen the scapular, shoulder, elbow, and wrist muscles that are involved in providing pulling forces. Integration of core and trunk muscle stabilization is an essential element of technique for many of these exercises. Pulling exercises are classified as general movement patterns, but some specific movement patterns that are used for isolating various pulling muscles to accomplish a variety of possible training goals are also included in this chapter. Upper body structure and function, along with specific muscle physiology and all biomechanical factors, were considered when developing the instructions for all elements of technique, such as alignment, positioning, motion, stabilization, and suggested breathing method.

These exercise selections vary in their difficulty of stabilization or movement demands in order to provide a well-balanced collection of movements to challenge individuals of all strength and fitness levels. Some exercises are more suited for addressing performance-based goals while others are ideal for achieving more aesthetic-based goals. Variations and modifications that will increase or decrease the level of challenge are also provided in the description section for many exercises. Consider the steps below when selecting exercises as they were derived through combining information relative to exercise technique presented in chapter 4 along with the exercise selection process presented in chapter 5 in order to help select and instruct the efficient performance of each exercise.

1. Identify the goal (aesthetic- or performance-based)
2. Select the desired movement pattern (general movement pattern or specific movement pattern)
3. Select the muscle groups to be targeted (muscle synergies or isolated muscles)
4. Identify alignment of the forces (pull of the muscles vs. pull or push of the resistance)
5. Consider the positioning options (proprioception vs. neural availability)
6. Focus on stabilization (more important than the actual movement)
7. Use and control the planned tempo (affects type of strength, is a component of volume)
8. Integrate breathing method or control

Machine Median Row

This exercise targets the lats and scapular retractors, and it works the rear deltoids and biceps as well. In addition, the direct pull of the resistance against the trunk challenges the spinal erectors and associated posterior trunk and core muscles. Rowing exercises are pulling movements that can be performed at different angles in the median plane. They provide maximal shortening of the lats and train the spinal and scapular muscles necessary for optimal posture. Therefore, rowing exercises can be good selections for both aesthetic- and performance-based goals. Proper posture and pelvic positioning is imperative for this exercise to prevent excessive stress on the lumbar spinal structures so be sure the individual has been instructed on proper technique.

Target Muscles

Latissimus dorsi, posterior deltoids, scapular retractors, spinal extensors

Joint Motions

Scapular retraction, shoulder extension, elbow flexion

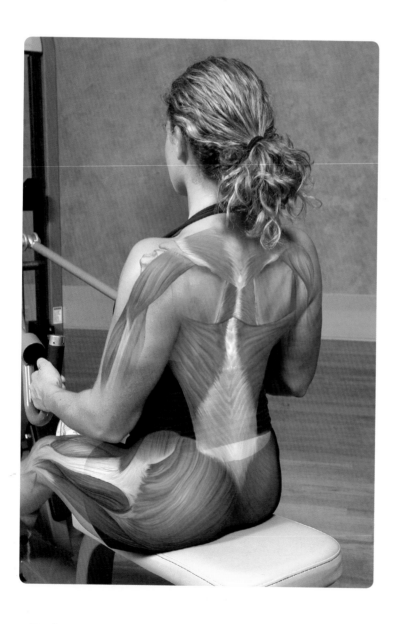

Alignment and Positioning

1. Grab the handles or a bar using a neutral grip with the hands parallel to the body.

2. Sit with the legs about shoulder-width apart and the knees bent as needed to allow for a natural arch in the lower back.

3. Begin with the arms straight, the scapula neutral to slightly protracted, and the spine in good posture. Then inhale.

Motion and Stabilization

1. Begin to exhale, activate the core, and start to pull the shoulder blades together while pulling the arms down and back.

2. Continue to retract the scapula, and pull the arms back until the elbows are aligned with the shoulders (or as far as possible) while maintaining proper posture.

3. Hold, slowly inhale, and allow the arms and scapula to be pulled back to the starting position while maintaining proper posture.

Trainer Techniques

1. Monitor spine and pelvic positioning, scapular, shoulder, and elbow motion

2. Cue scapular retractors, latissimus dorsi

3. Spot on the bar (assist or resist)

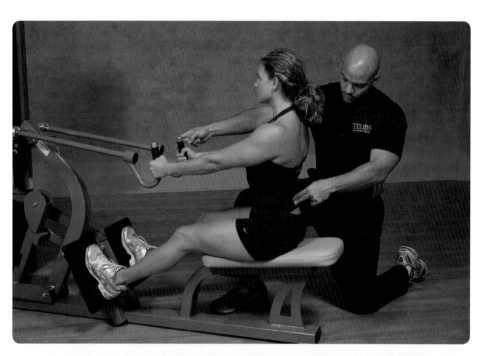

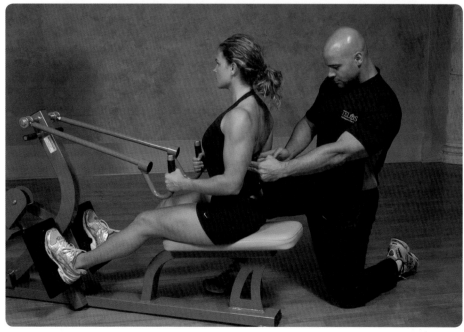

Dumbbell Median Row

This exercise targets the lats and scapular retractors, and it works the rear deltoids and biceps as well. In addition, the vertical pull of the resistance against the trunk places a high stabilization demand on the spinal and hip extensors. This and similar free weight exercises require a high level of hamstring flexibility in order to position the trunk in opposition to gravity and maintain a natural lumbar curvature. Using cable-pulley systems for standing rowing movements may be a better option if hip mobility and spinal stability are not yet adequate. One-arm braced or unbraced positions and alternate or piston movements are optional variations.

Target Muscles

Latissimus dorsi, posterior deltoids, scapular retractors, spinal extensors, hip extensors

Joint Motions

Scapular retraction, shoulder extension, elbow flexion

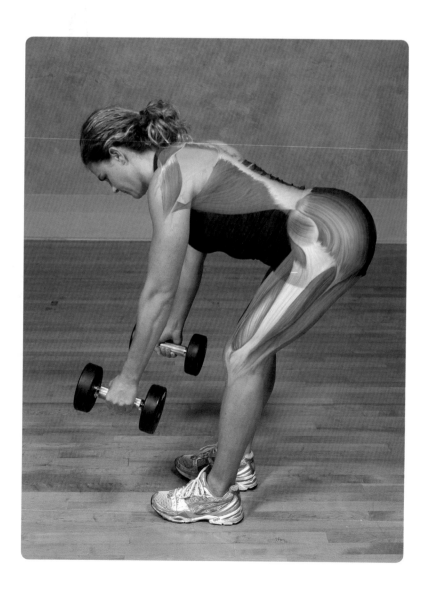

Alignment and Positioning

1. Hold the dumbbells with a neutral grip, and stand with the legs set just inside shoulder width.

2. Flex the hips, slightly bend the knees, and lean the upper body over until the trunk is close to parallel with the floor while maintaining good posture and a natural arch in the lower spine.

3. Begin with the dumbbells parallel to the body, the hands slightly in front of the shoulders, and the spine in good posture. Draw a deep breath.

Motion and Stabilization

1. Begin to exhale, activate the core, and start to pull the shoulder blades together while pulling the arms back and up.

2. Continue to retract the scapula and maintain posture. Pull the arms up and back, keeping the dumbbells outside the thighs, until the upper arms are about parallel to the body and the hands are under the navel.

3. Hold, slowly inhale, and allow the arms and scapula to be pulled back to the starting position while maintaining proper posture.

Trainer Techniques

1. Monitor spine and pelvic positioning, scapular, shoulder, and elbow motion

2. Cue scapular retractors, latissimus dorsi, possible contralateral glutes

3. Spot on forearm or on dumbbell

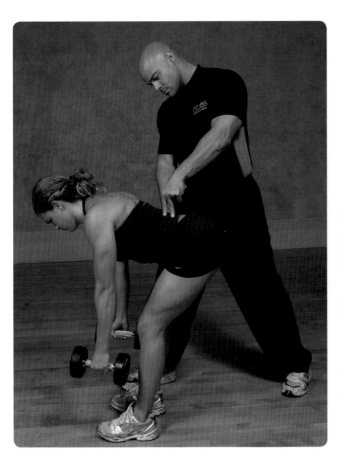
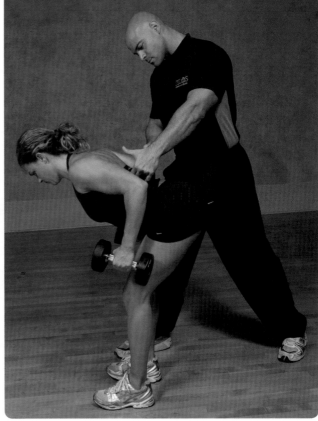

Cable One-Arm Median Row

This exercise targets the lats, scapular retractors, rear deltoids, and biceps. Pulling with one arm while in the lunge position also places a rotational force across the pelvis and spine that will require the glutes of the lead leg and other associated hip and trunk musculature of the posterior oblique subsystem (POS) for stabilization. This exercise is valuable for addressing performance-related goals such as improved pelvic-spinal stabilization, deceleration of rotational movements, and improved propulsion for walking, sprinting, or jumping. Mastering of this exercise should precede the Cable Trunk Rotation With Pull exercise presented in chapter 4.

Target Muscles

Posterior oblique subsystem (latissimus dorsi, contralateral gluteus maximus), teres major, posterior deltoids, scapular retractors, spinal extensors

Joint Motions

Scapular retraction, shoulder extension, elbow flexion

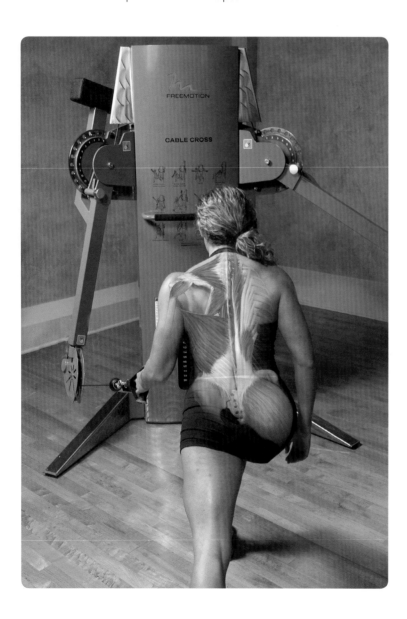

Cable One-Arm Median Row

Alignment and Positioning

1. Grasp the handle, then step back from the pulley into a lunge position, with the opposite leg forward and the legs about shoulder-width apart.

2. Begin with the arm aligned with the cable, the scapula slightly protracted, and the weight mostly on the lead leg.

3. Position the spine in good posture, and draw a deep breath.

Motion and Stabilization

1. Begin to exhale, activate the core, and start to retract the shoulder blade while pulling the arm back and up.

2. Continue to retract the scapula, and pull the arm up and the hand toward the navel until the upper arm is about parallel to the body.

3. Hold, slowly inhale, and allow the arm and scapula to be pulled back to the starting position while maintaining proper posture.

Trainer Techniques

1. Monitor spine and pelvic positioning, scapular, shoulder, and elbow motion

2. Cue scapular retractors, latissimus dorsi, possible contralateral glutes

3. Spot on forearm or on pelvic girdle

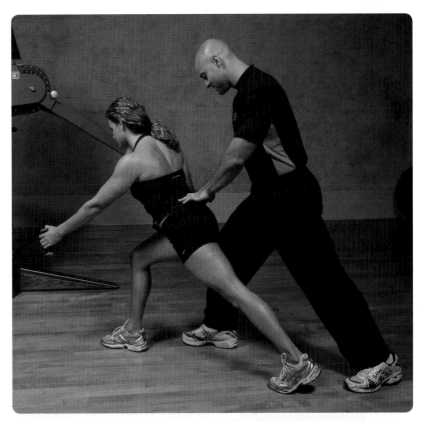

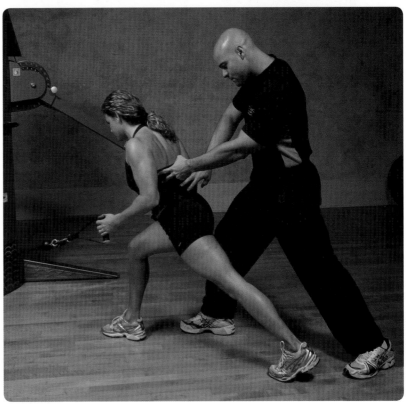

Cable Shoulder Extension

This exercise targets the lats and associated shoulder extensors. This isolated shoulder movement is a good selection for some people to better develop initial facilitation of the lats as opposed to rowing or pulling movements. Depending on the active shoulder flexion abilities of the lifter, this exercise can allow for high degrees of resisted shoulder movement because the starting position can be drastically varied. The standing position requires additional hip, core, and trunk musculature for stabilization and makes the use of heavy weight difficult. One-arm, lunge positions, one-leg, alternate movements, and piston movements are optional variations for this exercise.

Target Muscles

Latissimus dorsi, teres major, posterior deltoids, scapular depressors and retractors, spinal extensors

Joint Motions

Scapular depression, scapular retraction, shoulder extension

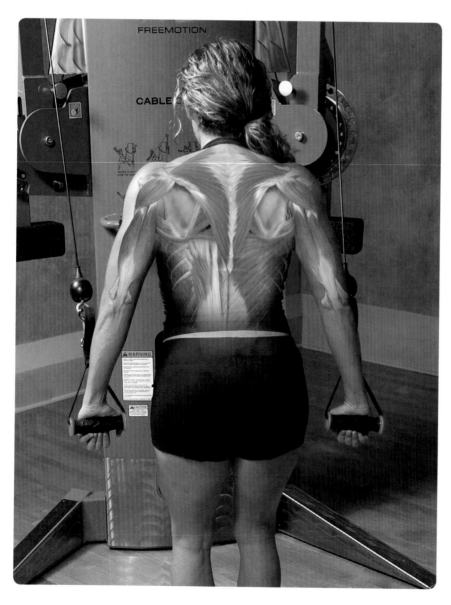

Cable Shoulder Extension

Alignment and Positioning

1. Hold the handles perpendicular to the body, then step back from the pulley with the legs about shoulder-width apart.

2. Begin with the hands just above the head, the arms straight, and the elbows slightly bent and pointed out.

3. Flex the hips and knees to position the trunk at about a 45-degree angle in good posture and with a natural arch in the lower spine. Draw a deep breath.

Motion and Stabilization

1. Begin to exhale, activate the core, and start to pull the shoulder blades down and together while pulling the arms down.

2. Continue to depress and retract the scapula, and pull the arms back as far as possible while maintaining proper posture.

3. Hold, slowly inhale, and allow the arms and scapula to be pulled back to the starting position while maintaining proper posture.

Trainer Techniques

1. Monitor spine and pelvic positioning, scapular and shoulder motion

2. Cue scapular depressors and retractors, latissimus dorsi

3. Spot on forearms

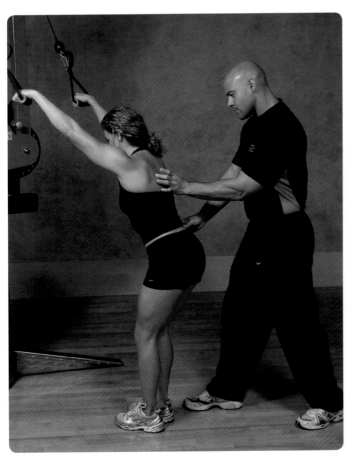
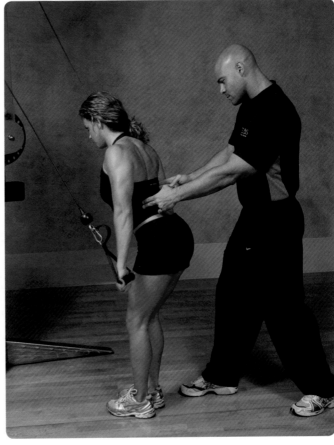

Machine Frontal Pull-Up

Pulling exercises in the frontal plane require substantially more difficult scapular-thoracic and scapular-humeral rhythm than rowing exercises performed in the median plane require. This exercise still targets the lats but will also demand more from the rhomboids and other scapular downward rotators and scapular depressors. The ability to produce optimal posture, particularly in the thoracic spine, is a prerequisite for optimal frontal plane scapular movement. Frontal plane pulling with a bar forces a closed-chain action of the arms that can be stressful to the structures of the shoulder, elbow, and wrist joints. Proper hand placement and technique are imperative in order to decrease these risks so be sure the lifter has been instructed on proper technique and hand placement.

Target Muscles

Latissimus dorsi, teres major, posterior deltoids, scapular depressors, rhomboids, biceps

Joint Motions

Scapular depression, scapular downward rotation, shoulder frontal extension (adduction), elbow flexion

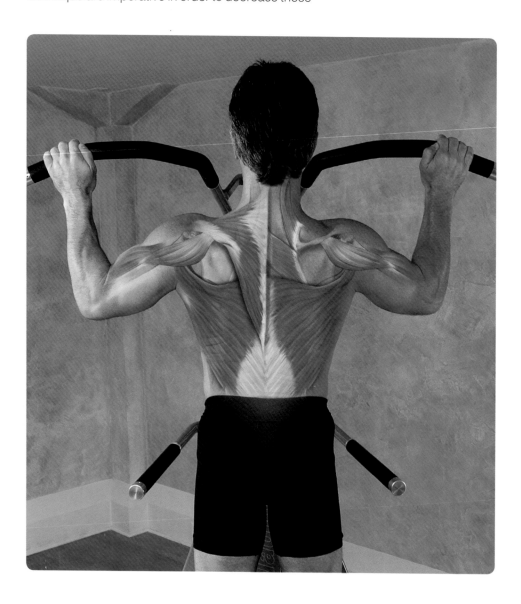

Machine Frontal Pull-Up

Alignment and Positioning

1. Grasp the bar with the hands outside shoulder width so that a 90-degree angle may be formed at the elbow as you pull up.

2. Begin with the knees on the pad if assistance is desired, with the arms straight, the elbows pointed out, and the scapula elevated.

3. Position the spine in good posture with the chest up, and draw a deep breath.

Motion and Stabilization

1. Begin to exhale, activate the core, and start to pull the shoulder blades down while pulling the elbows out and the body straight up between the hands.

2. Continue to depress and rotate the scapula downward. Pull the body up while keeping good posture and keeping the scapula depressed.

3. Hold, slowly inhale, and allow the body to lower and the scapula to return to the starting position while maintaining proper posture.

Trainer Techniques

1. Monitor spine and pelvic positioning, scapular and shoulder motion

2. Cue scapular depressors and retractors, latissimus dorsi

3. Spot under rib cage or on machine pad

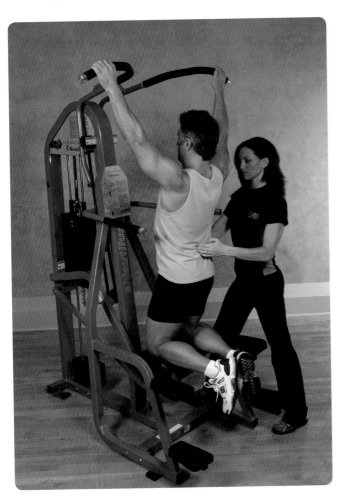
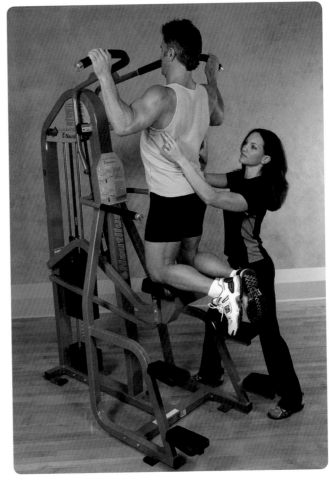

Cable One-Arm Frontal Pull-Down

Pulling movements in the frontal plane require a more difficult scapular-thoracic and scapular-humeral rhythm than rowing movements that occur in the median plane require. This open-chain pulling movement allows for independent scapular and arm movement, which requires more scapular and shoulder control and can reduce some of the potentially destructive forces associated with closed-chain options. The one-arm movement while in a lunge position requires more assistance from the posterior oblique subsystem (POS) and other hip, core, and trunk muscles for stabilization than the seated, two-arm variations require. Lat pull-downs can also be performed with alternate or piston movements for varied training effects.

Target Muscles

Posterior oblique subsystem (latissimus dorsi, contralateral gluteus maximus), teres major, posterior deltoids, scapular depressors, rhomboids, biceps

Joint Motions

Scapular depression, scapular downward rotation, shoulder frontal extension (adduction), elbow flexion

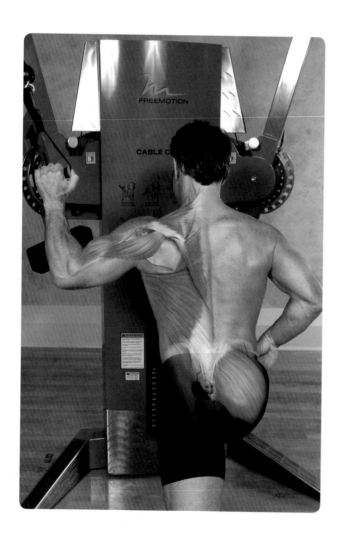

Cable One-Arm Frontal Pull-Down

Alignment and Positioning

1. Grasp the handle, then step back from the pulley into a lunge position, with the opposite leg forward and the legs about shoulder-width apart.

2. Begin with a natural arch in the lower spine, the arm straight, the elbow out, and the scapula rotated upward.

3. Position the trunk in good posture and in direct alignment with the cable. Slightly lift the chest up, and draw a deep breath.

Motion and Stabilization

1. Begin to exhale, activate the core, and start to pull the shoulder blade downward while keeping the elbow out as it flexes.

2. Continue to depress and rotate the scapula downward. Pull the arm down while keeping the hand away from the body and the upper arm and trunk in alignment with the cable.

3. Hold, slowly inhale, and allow the arm and scapula to be pulled out and up to the starting position while maintaining proper posture.

Trainer Techniques

1. Monitor spine and pelvic positioning, scapular, shoulder, and elbow motion

2. Cue scapular depressors and retractors, latissimus dorsi

3. Spot on upper forearm

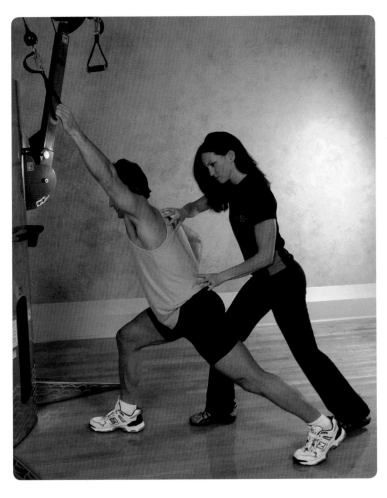

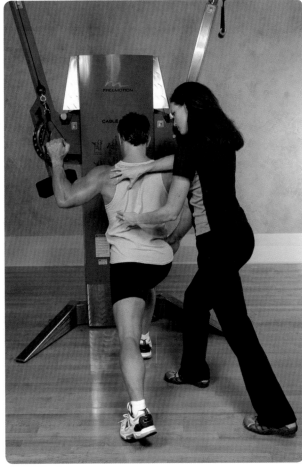

Dumbbell Horizontal Row

This exercise targets the posterior deltoids and also works the scapular retractors, shoulder external rotators, and biceps. In addition, the vertical pull of the resistance directly challenges the spinal erectors and hip extensors for trunk and pelvic stability. Although lifting free weights while standing has more transference to life situations, these types of exercises require a high level of hamstring flexibility in order to align the body properly against gravity. Using cable-pulley systems may be a better option for some people until appropriate hip mobility and spinal stability are achieved.

Target Muscles

Posterior deltoids, shoulder external rotators, scapular retractors, spinal extensors, hip extensors

Joint Motions

Scapular retraction, shoulder horizontal extension, elbow flexion

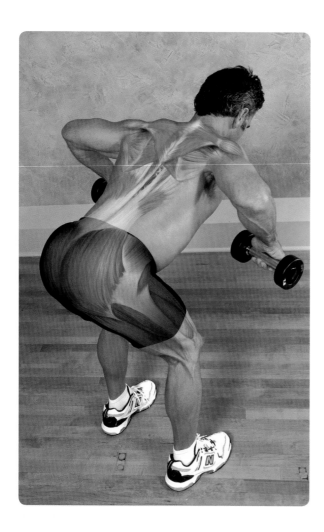

Dumbbell Horizontal Row

Alignment and Positioning

1. Hold the dumbbells with a neutral grip, and stand with the legs set outside shoulder width.

2. Flex the hips, slightly bend the knees, and lean the upper body over until the trunk is close to parallel with the floor. Maintain good posture and a natural arch in the lower spine.

3. Begin with the dumbbells perpendicular to the body, the hands straight down from the shoulders, and the spine in good posture. Draw a deep breath.

Motion and Stabilization

1. Begin to exhale, activate the core, and start to pull the shoulder blades together while pulling the arms out and up.

2. Continue to retract the scapula and maintain posture. Pull the arms out and up until the upper arms are about parallel to the floor, with the elbows straight out from the shoulders.

3. Hold, slowly inhale, and allow the arms and scapula to be pulled back to the starting position while maintaining proper posture.

Trainer Techniques

1. Monitor spine and pelvic positioning, scapular, shoulder, and elbow motion

2. Cue scapular retractors, posterior deltoids

3. Spot on upper forearms

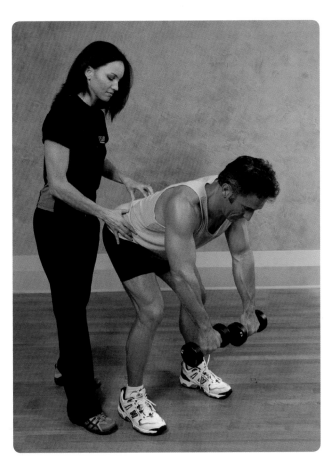 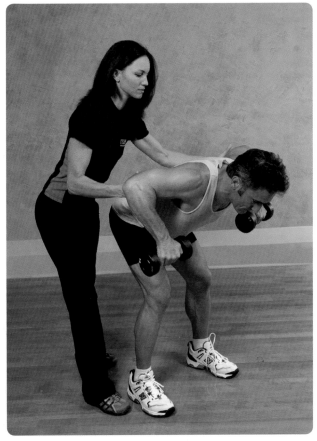

Cable One-Arm Horizontal Row

This exercise targets the posterior deltoids but also works the scapular retractors, shoulder external rotators, and biceps. The one-arm, standing option has higher stabilization demands that will require more involvement of the posterior oblique subsystem (POS) and associated hip, core, and trunk muscles than the two-arm, seated options require. Exercises performed while standing may be more transferable to most life situations, but maximal loads are difficult because there is no use of an external anchor. For varied training effects, this exercise can be performed seated, kneeling, with two arms, or with alternate or piston arm movements.

Target Muscles

Posterior deltoids, shoulder external rotators, scapular retractors, spinal extensors, hip extensors, posterior oblique subsystem

Joint Motions

Scapular retraction, shoulder horizontal extension, elbow flexion

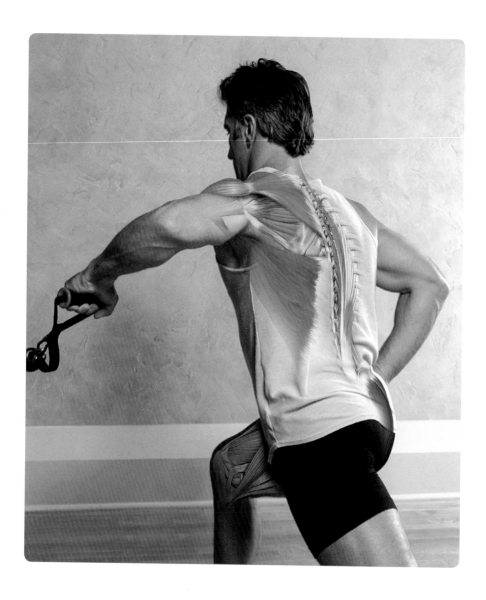

Cable One-Arm Horizontal Row

Alignment and Positioning

1. Grasp the handle, then step back from the pulley into a lunge position with the opposite leg forward and with the legs about shoulder-width apart.

2. Begin with the arm aligned with the cable, the elbow pointed out, the scapula slightly protracted, and the weight mostly over the lead leg.

3. Position the spine in good posture, and draw a deep breath.

Motion and Stabilization

1. Begin to exhale, activate the core, and start to retract the shoulder blade while pulling the arm out and back.

2. Continue to retract the scapula and maintain posture. Pull the arm out and back until the elbow is about parallel to the shoulder, keeping the upper arm parallel to the floor.

3. Hold, slowly inhale, and allow the arm and scapula to be pulled back to the starting position while maintaining proper posture.

Trainer Techniques

1. Monitor spine and pelvic positioning, scapular, shoulder, and elbow motion

2. Cue scapular retractors, posterior deltoid

3. Spot on upper forearm or possibly pelvic girdle or ribcage

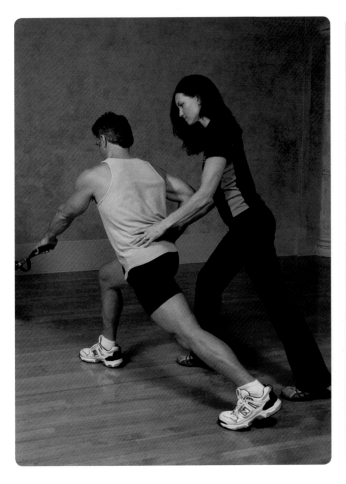 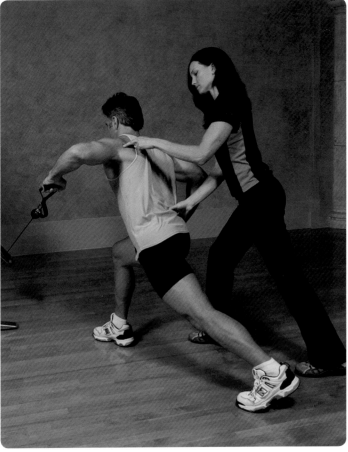

Barbell Scapular Elevation (Shrug)

This exercise targets the scapula elevators and upper back and neck extensors. This exercise could have been included in pushing movements as well, because the trapezius (one of the targeted muscles) is primarily responsible for upward rotation of the scapula, which is necessary for overhead pushing movements. The technique presented for this exercise contains important modifications to the traditional "shrug" movement and can help to prepare scapular and upper spinal muscles for power training exercises, such as the modified clean or hang clean. Notice that the trunk is positioned in a forward lean at the hips. This alignment allows for greater trapezius and scapular retractor involvement, which consequently helps to decrease the load on the levator scapula muscles and reduce stress on the cervical spine.

Target Muscles

Upper and mid trapezius, levator scapula, cervical and upper spinal extensors

Joint Motions

Scapular elevation and retraction

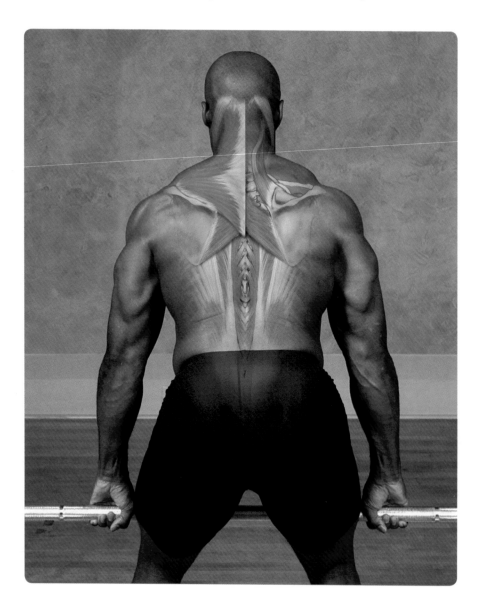

Barbell Scapular Elevation (Shrug)

Alignment and Positioning

1. Stand in good posture with the feet directly under the hips. Grasp the bar using an overhand grip, with the hands just outside shoulder width.

2. Draw a deep breath, flex the hips and knees slightly, and begin to push the hips back and lean the trunk forward.

3. Position the spine at an approximate 45-degree angle, with good posture and a natural arch in the lower spine, and with the bar close to the thighs.

Motion and Stabilization

1. Begin to exhale, activate the core, and start to pull the shoulder blades up and together while keeping the arms relaxed.

2. Continue to elevate and retract the scapula, lifting the arms and weight while pushing the chest out to improve posture.

3. Hold, then slowly inhale and allow the arms and scapula to be pulled back to the starting position while maintaining posture.

Trainer Techniques

1. Monitor spine and pelvic positioning, scapular motion

2. Cue scapular elevators and retractors

3. Spot on upper arms

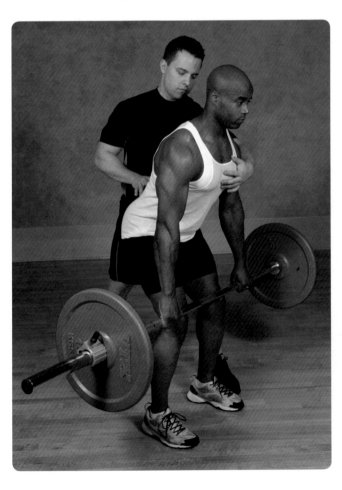
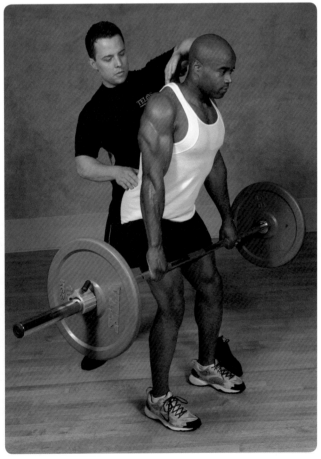

Cable Shoulder External Rotation

This exercise targets the posterior rotator cuff muscles. A similar exercise that trains internal rotation of the shoulder could be performed to target the subscapularis. Although strengthening the entire rotator cuff musculature would be advised, it is the external rotators that tend to become weak with faulty postural adaptations and are also more prone to injury. This is because the external rotators have less support from larger muscles than the internal rotators do. The external rotators are also required for deceleration of the arm during any throwing or swinging movements, leaving them at high risk for injury. Strong rotator cuff muscles should be considered a prerequisite for ballistic exercises such as cleans or snatches.

Target Muscles

Infraspinatus, teres minor

Joint Motions

Shoulder external rotation

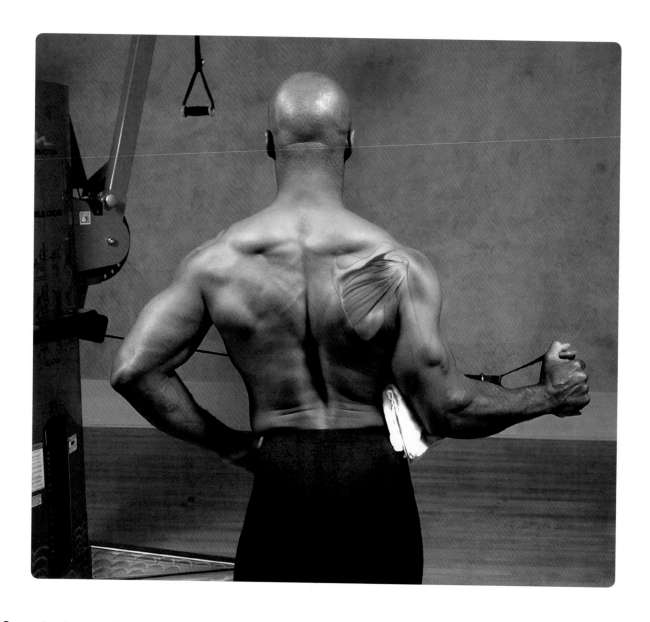

Cable Shoulder External Rotation

Alignment and Positioning

1. Stand in good posture, and set the adjustable pulley at elbow height with a single-handle attachment.

2. Place a rolled towel under the elbow to abduct the upper arm about 10 to 20 degrees, and flex the elbow to 90 degrees.

3. Begin with the arm internally rotated. Stabilize the scapula and draw a deep breath.

Motion and Stabilization

1. Begin to exhale, activate the core, and start to rotate the shoulder, pulling the arm out and across the body and keeping the elbow fixed.

2. Continue to pull the arm out, keeping the wrist neutral and the elbow pressed against the towel. Maintain good posture and a stable scapula.

3. Hold, slowly inhale, and allow the arm to be pulled back to the starting position while maintaining elbow, scapular, and postural positioning.

Trainer Techniques

1. Monitor spine and pelvic positioning, scapular motion

2. Cue shoulder external rotators

3. Spot on forearm or wrist

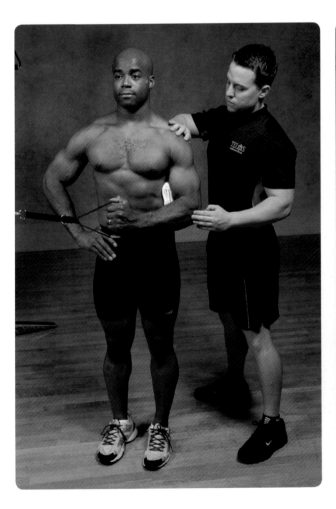
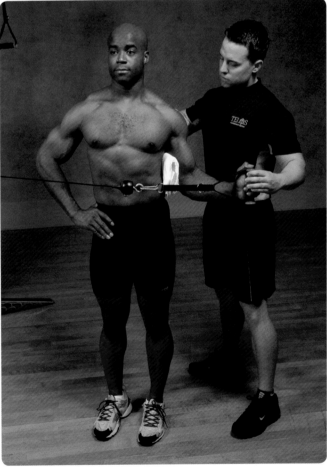

Dumbbell Shoulder External Rotation

This exercise targets combined strengthening of the shoulder abductors and posterior rotator cuff muscles. The arm is positioned below 90 degrees of abduction. This position better targets different fibers of the infraspinatus, provides a stabilization demand for the deltoid muscles, and allows for full external rotation with less chance of impingement than when in higher positions of shoulder abduction. The elbow is held at 80 degrees, and an isolated movement is performed to ensure specific targeting of the external rotators. Having the lifter work in a standing position and using free weights make this exercise more transferable to life situations. Strengthening the rotator cuff should be considered a prerequisite for ballistic movements such as cleans or snatches.

Target Muscles

Infraspinatus, teres minor, deltoids, scapular stabilizers

Joint Motions

Shoulder external rotation

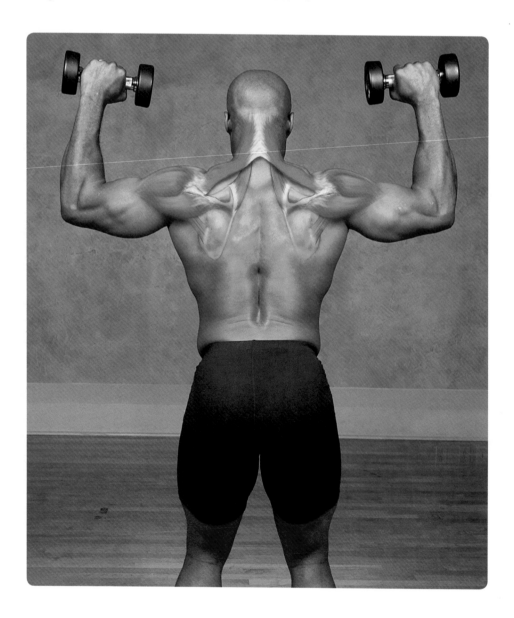

Dumbbell Shoulder External Rotation

Alignment and Positioning

1. Stand in good posture, with the hips and knees slightly flexed and the trunk in a forward lean.

2. Abduct the arms to about 80 degrees, with the elbows bent at 90 degrees, keeping the wrists neutral. Position the lower arms and the dumbbells about parallel to the floor.

3. Stabilize the spine and shoulders, then draw a deep breath.

Motion and Stabilization

1. Begin to exhale, activate the core, and start to rotate the shoulders, pulling the lower arms and the dumbbells up while keeping the wrists straight.

2. Continue to rotate the shoulders and pull the arms up as far as possible, keeping the forward lean of the trunk with the spine in good posture and the upper arms at about 80 degrees.

3. Hold, then slowly inhale and allow the arms and dumbbells to lower to the starting position while maintaining posture and shoulder positioning.

Trainer Techniques

1. Monitor spine and pelvic positioning, shoulder motion

2. Cue shoulder external rotators

3. Spot under forearms or possibly by slightly bracing under upper arms

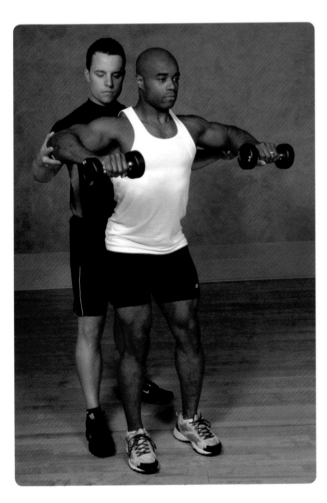
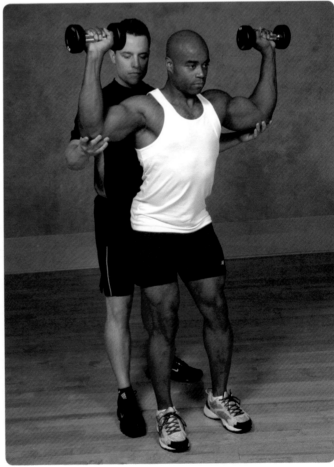

Dumbbell 15-Degree Elbow Flexion With Supination

This exercise targets the full action of the elbow flexors. Although isolated elbow flexion is often selected for aesthetic-based goals, the technique presented here requires significant levels of stabilization demand for scapular depressors and retractors, so it may help improve postural abilities as well as develop the biceps. The offset position of the dumbbells further challenges supination, and the slight initial shoulder flexion helps to promote scapular actions that are associated with good posture. Variations of this exercise include maintaining the elbows in a neutral position to target the brachioradialis, or in supinated positions to better target the biceps brachii.

Target Muscles

Biceps group, wrist flexors, shoulder and scapular stabilizers

Joint Motions

Slight shoulder flexion, elbow flexion, radioulnar supination

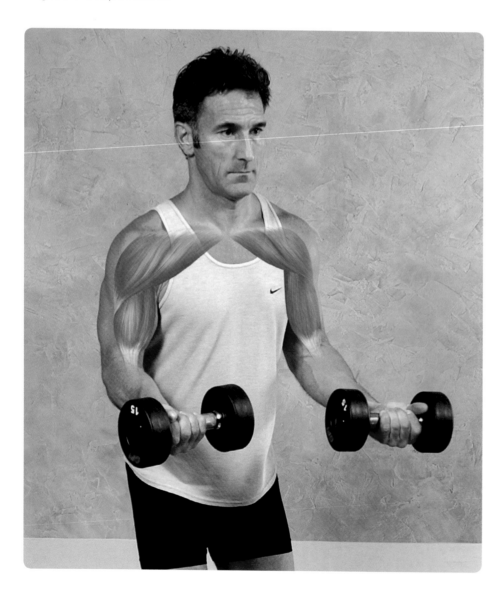

Dumbbell 15-Degree Elbow Flexion With Supination

Alignment and Positioning

1. Stand with the hips and knees slightly flexed, and hold a set of dumbbells, with the lower arms in a neutral position.

2. Slightly retract the shoulder blades, and position the spine in good posture. Slide the hands all the way forward on the handles of the dumbbells to unbalance the load.

3. Begin with the hands and dumbbells straight down from the shoulders, with the elbows slightly bent. Draw a deep breath.

Motion and Stabilization

1. Begin to exhale, activate the core, and slightly flex the shoulders to begin pulling the arms forward while also flexing the elbows.

2. Continue to flex the elbows, and begin supinating the lower arms, causing the dumbbells to twist as they are pulled forward and up as far as possible. Maintain scapular and trunk positioning.

3. Hold, then slowly inhale and allow the arms to slowly lower and twist back to the starting position while maintaining proper posture.

Trainer Techniques

1. Monitor spine, pelvic, and scapular positioning, shoulder and elbow movement

2. Cue biceps group

3. Spot under forearms or on wrists

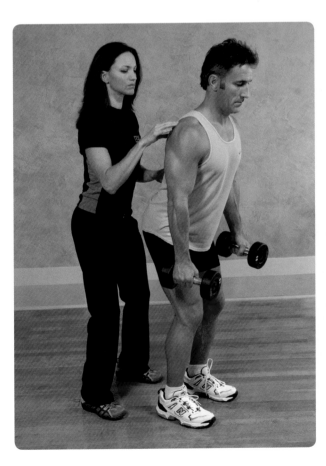 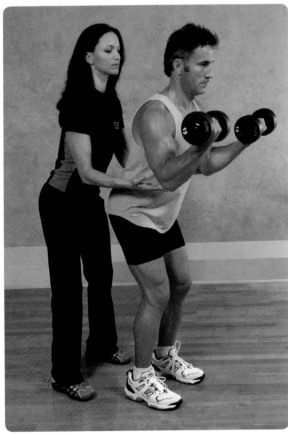

Cable One-Arm 90-Degree Elbow Flexion

This exercise targets the biceps group. It emphasizes the short head of the biceps by preshortening the long-head biceps, which causes it to become somewhat active insufficient. The shoulder positioning used in this exercise also creates different scapular and shoulder stabilization demands than lower angles do. If using a barbell as opposed to separate handles, it is important to have the lifter grasp the bar with the natural carrying angle in place to decrease some of the additional shearing forces associated with most closed-chain upper body exercises. Individual handles also allow two-hand, alternate, and piston movements for varied training effects.

Target Muscles

Biceps group, wrist flexors, shoulder and scapular stabilizers

Joint Motions

Slight shoulder flexion, elbow flexion

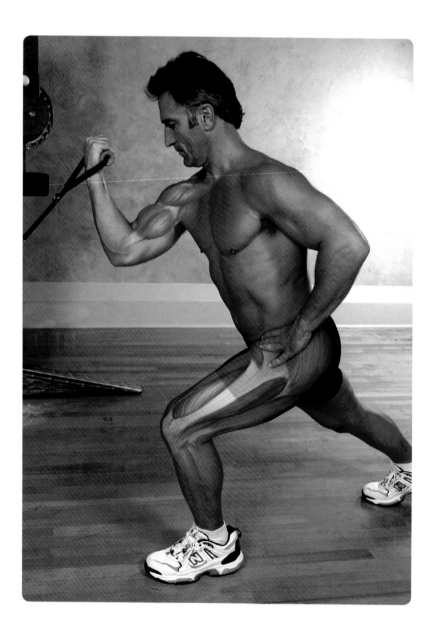

Cable One-Arm 90-Degree Elbow Flexion

Alignment and Positioning

1. Stand with the hips and knees slightly flexed, and grasp the handle of the upper cable in a supinated position.

2. Pull the shoulder blades slightly together, slightly lift the chest, and position the spine in good posture.

3. Position the arm in line with the cable pulley, and begin with tension on the biceps. Draw a deep breath.

Motion and Stabilization

1. Begin to exhale, activate the core, slightly flex the shoulder, and begin to pull the arm up while flexing the elbow.

2. Continue to pull the lower arm up and back as far as possible while maintaining scapular, shoulder, wrist, and postural positioning.

3. Hold, then slowly inhale and allow the arm to be slowly pulled back to the starting position while maintaining proper posture.

Trainer Techniques

1. Monitor spine, pelvic, and scapular positioning, shoulder and elbow movement

2. Cue biceps group

3. Spot under forearm or possibly on pelvic girdle or rib cage

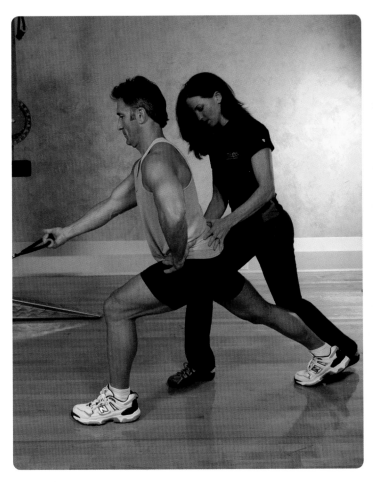
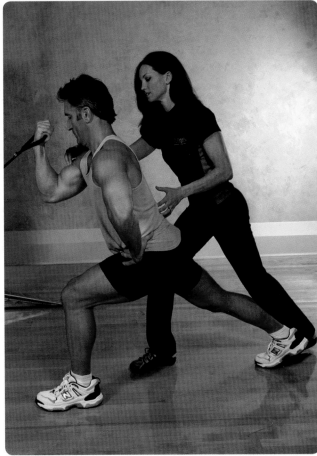

Bibliography

Aaberg, E. 2000. *Resistance training instruction.* Champaign, IL: Human Kinetics.

Aaberg, E. 2001. *Resistance training instruction video series: The lower body.* Champaign, IL: Human Kinetics.

Aaberg, E. 2001. *Resistance training instruction video series: The trunk.* Champaign, IL: Human Kinetics.

Aaberg, E. 2001. *Resistance training instruction video series: The upper body.* Champaign, IL: Human Kinetics.

Alter, M. 1996. *Science of flexibility.* 2nd ed. Champaign, IL: Human Kinetics.

Bompa, T., and L. Cornacchia. 1998. *Serious strength training.* Champaign, IL: Human Kinetics.

Brown, L., V. Ferrigno, and J.C. Santana. 2000. *Training for speed, agility, and quickness.* Champaign, IL: Human Kinetics.

Calais-Germain, B. 1993. *Anatomy of movement.* Seattle: Eastland Press.

Check, P. 1995. *Program design.* Encinitas, CA: C.H.E.K. Institute.

Check, P. 1995. *Scientific back training.* Encinitas, CA: C.H.E.K. Institute.

Check, P. 1996. *Dynamic medicine ball training.* Video and correspondence course. Encinitas, CA: C.H.E.K. Institute.

Check, P. 1998. *Golf conditioning.* Encinitas, CA: C.H.E.K. Institute.

Check, P. 1998. *Scientific core training.* Video and correspondence course. Encinitas, CA: C.H.E.K. Institute.

Check, P. 1999. *The outer unit.* ptonthenet.com: Personal Training on the Net.

Check, P. 2000. *Movement that matters.* Encinitas, CA: C.H.E.K. Institute.

Chu, D. 1992. *Jumping into plyometrics.* Champaign, IL: Leisure Press.

Clark, M. 2001. *Integrated training for the new millennium.* Thousand Oaks, CA: National Academy of Sports Medicine.

Enoka, R. 2002. *Neuromechanics of human movement.* 3rd ed. Champaign, IL: Human Kinetics.

Fleck, S., and W. Kraemer. 1997. *Designing resistance training programs.* 2nd ed. Champaign, IL: Human Kinetics.

Fleck, S., and W. Kraemer. 1996. *Periodization breakthrough.* Ronkonkoma, NY: Advanced Research Press.

Foran, B. 2001. *High-performance sports conditioning.* Champaign, IL: Human Kinetics.

Heyward, V. 1998. *Advanced fitness assessment and exercise prescription.* 3rd ed. Champaign, IL: Human Kinetics.

Lephart, S., and F. Fu. 2000. *Proprioception and neuromuscular control in joint stability.* Champaign, IL: Human Kinetics.

National Strength and Conditioning Association. 1994. *Essentials of strength and conditioning,* ed. by T. Baechle and R. Earle. Champaign, IL: Human Kinetics.

Norkin, C., and P. Levangie. 1992. *Joint structure and function a comprehensive analysis.* Philadelphia: F.A. Davis.

Poliquin, C. 1997. *The Poliquin principles.* Napa, CA: Dayton Writers Group.

Poliquin, C. 1998. *Charles Poliquin's advanced strength training certification program.* Napa, CA: Dayton.

Purvis, T. 1995. *Focus on fitness.* Instructor video series. Oklahoma City: Focus on Fitness.

Purvis, T. 1997. *Resistance training specialist.* The Mastery Course Manual 1. Oklahoma City: Focus on Fitness.

Purvis, T. 1997. *Resistance training specialist.* The Mastery Course Manual 2. Oklahoma City: Focus on Fitness.

Purvis, T. 1997. *Resistance training specialist.* The Mastery Course Manual 3. Oklahoma City: Focus on Fitness.

Purvis, T. 1997. *Resistance training specialist.* The Mastery Course Manual 4. Oklahoma City: Focus on Fitness.

Radcliffe, J., and R. Farentinos. 1999. *High-powered plyometrics.* Champaign, IL: Human Kinetics.

Renstrom, P.A.F.H. 1993. *Sports injuries: Basic principles of prevention and care.* Oxford: Blackwell Scientific.

Richardson, C., G. Jull, P. Hodges, and J. Hides. 1999. *Therapeutic exercise for spinal segmental stabilization in low back pain.* London: Churchill Livingstone.

Schmidt, R.H., and C.A. Wrisberg. 1991. *Motor learning and performance.* Champaign, IL: Human Kinetics.

Siff, M. 1998. *Facts and fallacies of fitness.* 2nd ed. Johannesburg, South Africa: Author.

Siff, M. 2000. *Supertraining.* 5th ed. Denver: Supertraining Institute.

Vleeming, A., V. Mooney, T. Dorman, C. Snijders, and R. Stoeckart. 1997. *Movement, stability and low back pain.* New York: Churchill Livingstone.

Watkins, J. 1999. *Structure and function of the musculoskeletal system.* Champaign, IL: Human Kinetics.

Index

Page numbers followed by an *f* or a *t* indicate a figure or table, respectively.

A

acceleration 43
active system
 actions and roles of muscles 12-13
 muscle structure 8, 9-10*f*, 11
 muscular subsystems 13
 overview 8, 9*f*
aesthetic-based goals 68
agility 48-49
agonist muscles 12-13
alignment 56-57
alpha motor neurons 15
anatomical design and function
 general movement patterns 18
 neuromuscular efficiency 17-18
 systems involved. *See* active system;
  control system; passive system
ankle
 dumbbell one-leg ankle extension
  188-189
 frontal plane movement 24*f*
 machine ankle flexion 194-195
 machine bent-leg ankle extension
  192-193
 machine straight-leg ankle extension
  190-191
 median plane movement 21*f*
antagonist muscles 12-13
anterior oblique subsystem (AOS) 79
appendicular skeleton 6
arms. *See* upper-body exercises
articular cartilage 7
axial skeleton 6

B

back. *See* upper-body exercises
balance 35-36, 60-61
barbell-based exercises
 hang clean 160-161
 hip extension 172-173
 horizontal press 200-201
 scapular elevation 236-237
 squat 148-149
basal ganglia 17
bent-leg raises 112-113
biomotor abilities improvement
 agility 48-49
 endurance 33-34
 mobility. *See* mobility
 muscle hypertrophy and 49-51
 power 45-48
 speed and. *See* speed
 stability 34-36
 strength and. *See* strength
brain stem 16
breathing 63-65

C

cable-based exercises
 hip abduction 176-177
 hip adduction 178-179
 knee extension 180-181
 knee flexion 184-185

one-arm 90-degree elbow extension
 214-215
one-arm 90-degree elbow flexion
 244-245
one-arm decline horizontal press
 204-205
one-arm frontal pull-down 230-231
one-arm horizontal row 235
one-arm median row 224-225
shoulder extension 226-227
shoulder external rotation 238-239
trunk rotation with flexion 132-133
trunk rotation with press 136-137
trunk rotation with pull 134-135
zero-degree elbow extension 216-
 217
cartilage 7
cartilaginous joints 6
cerebellum 16-17
cerebral cortex 17
compound lower-body exercises
 balance squat 142-143
 barbell hang clean 160-161
 barbell squat 148-149
 body weight squat 140-141
 body weight stationary lunge 152-153
 dumbbell deadlift 144-145, 145
 dumbbell reverse lunge 154-155
 dumbbell side lunge 156-157
 dumbbell snatch 162-163
 machine seated leg press 150-151
 med ball traveling lunge 158-159
 narrow-stance squat 146-147
 steps when selecting exercises 139
 wide-stance squat 144-145
concentric contraction 11
connective tissue 6-7, 38-39
control system
 cerebral cortex 17
 lower brain 16-17
 overview 14, 15*f*
 spinal cord 15-16
coordination and motor control 18
core exercises
 bent-leg raises 112-113
 four-point core activation 108-109
 quadraplex 110-111
 steps when selecting 107
curvilinear motion 55
cycles, program 91

D

deep longitudinal subsystem (DLS) 78
dumbbell-based exercises
 15-degree elbow flexion 242-243
 deadlift 144-145, 145
 frontal press 210-211
 horizontal press 198-199
 horizontal row 232-233
 incline median press 208-209
 median row 222-223
 one-arm/one-leg frontal press 212-
  213

one-leg ankle extension 188-189
one-leg hip extension 174-175
reverse lunge 154-155
shoulder external rotation 240-241
side lunge 156-157
snatch 162-163
swiss ball one-arm horizontal press
 202-203
duration and volume 88

E

eccentric contraction 11
elbow
 cable one-arm 90-degree elbow
  extension 214-215
 cable one-arm 90-degree elbow
  flexion 244-245
 cable zero-degree elbow extension
  216-217
 dumbbell 15-degree elbow flexion
  242-243
 median plane movement 23*f*
endurance 33-34
exercise motion 55-56
exercise selection. *See also specific
 types of exercises*
 goals determination 67-68
 risks versus benefits determination
  80
 system of naming exercises 106
 targeting desired movements. *See*
  general movement patterns
 targeting desired muscle groups. *See*
  muscles
exhalation 77

F

fast-twitch muscle fibers 41, 42
fat loss and hypertrophy 49-51
fibrocartilage 7
fibrous joints 6
flexibility deficit 37
four-point core activation 108-109
frequency and volume 88-89
frontal plane movement 24-26*f*
full-body routines 93-94, 96-99*t*

G

gait patterns 74-75
gamma motor neurons 15-16
general movement patterns
 gait patterns 74-75
 overview 68-70
 pulling patterns 72-73
 pushing patterns 72, 73*f*
 spinal extension 71
 spinal flexion 70
 squat patterns 73-74
 trunk rotation 71, 72*f*
general plane motion 55
genetics and strength 31
goal identification 54-55
Golgi tendon organs (GTOs) 16

H

half ball trunk lateral flexion 126-127
hip
    barbell hip extension 172-173
    braced one-leg hip flexion 166-167
    cable hip abduction 176-177
    cable hip adduction 178-179
    dumbbell one-leg hip extension 174-175
    45-degree hip extension 170-171
    frontal plane movement 24f
    horizontal plane movement 27f
    median plane movement 22f
    swiss ball double-leg hip flexion 168-169
horizontal plane movement 27-28f
hyaline 7
hypertrophy 49-51, 84

I

incline bench exercises
    reverse trunk flexion 118-119
    trunk extension 122-123
    trunk flexion 114-115
inhalation 76-77
inner unit (core) 76-77
intensity
    defined 83
    duration and frequency and 84-85
    recovery and 85
    sequence and 85
    volume and 83-84
isolated lower-body exercises
    barbell hip extension 172-173
    braced one-leg hip flexion 166-167
    cable hip abduction 176-177
    cable hip adduction 178-179
    cable knee extension 180-181
    cable knee flexion 184-185
    dumbbell one-leg ankle extension 188-189
    dumbbell one-leg hip extension 174-175
    45-degree hip extension 170-171
    machine ankle flexion 194-195
    machine bent-leg ankle extension 192-193
    machine knee extension 182-183
    machine knee flexion 186-187
    machine straight-leg ankle extension 190-191
    steps when selecting exercises 165
    swiss ball double-leg hip flexion 168-169
isometric contraction 11

J

joint capsules 7
joint mechanics
    frontal plane movement 24-26f
    horizontal plane movement 27-28f
    median plane movement 21-23f
    planes of motion 20f
joints 6, 7f
Jones, Arthur 63
Jumping Into Plyometrics 46, 47

K

King, Ian 63
knee
    cable knee extension 180-181
    cable knee flexion 184-185
    horizontal plane movement 27f
    machine knee extension 182-183
    machine knee flexion 186-187
    median plane movement 21f

L

lactic acid 33-34
lateral subsystem (LS) 78
leg exercises. *See* compound lower-body exercises; isolated lower-body exercises
ligaments 7
linear motion 55
lower-body exercises. *See* compound lower-body exercises; isolated lower-body exercises
lower brain 16-17
lunges
    body weight stationary 152-153
    dumbbell reverse 154-155
    dumbbell side 156-157
    med ball traveling 158-159

M

machine-based exercises
    ankle flexion 194-195
    bent-leg ankle extension 192-193
    frontal pull-up 228-229
    knee extension 182-183
    knee flexion 186-187
    median row 220-221
    seated leg press 150-151
    straight-leg ankle extension 190-191
    trunk rotation 130-131
maximal oxygen consumption ($\dot{V}O_2max$) 33
median plane movement 21-23f
mobility
    connective tissue limits 38-39
    described 36-37
    muscle limits 37-38
    planes of motion 55
    sensorimotor system 39
    skeletal limits 38
    speed and 43-44
    stretching and 39-41
motion. *See* range of motion (ROM)
Motor Learning and Performance 18
muscles
    actions and roles 12-13
    anterior oblique subsystem 79
    basic structure 8, 9-11f, 11
    deep longitudinal subsystem 78
    hypertrophy and 49-51
    inner unit (core) 76-77
    isolation of specific 80
    lateral subsystem 78
    mobility and 37-38
    posterior oblique subsystem 79
    size relation to strength 31
    subsystems 13
muscle spindles 16
myotatic stretch reflex 46

N

naming of exercises 106
neck
    frontal plane movement 26f
    horizontal plane movement 28f
    median plane movement 23f
neutralizer muscles 13

O

onset of blood lactate accumulation (OBLA) 33-34
osteoarthritis 7

P

passive system
    connective tissue 6-7
    joints 6, 7f
    skeleton 4, 5f, 6

pelvic positioning 59f
performance-based goals 68
periodization and program design 90-93
phases, training 91-93
planes of motion 20f
plyometric training 46, 47f, 48
Poliquin, Charles 63
Poliquin Principles, The 63
positioning of the spine 57
posterior oblique subsystem (POS) 79
posture 58, 59f
power
    overview 45-46
    plyometric training 46, 47f, 48
presses. *See* upper-body pushing exercises
program design
    intensity 83-85
    periodization and 90-93
    recovery 89
    routines versus programs 81-82
    sample routines 93-94, 96-103t
    sequence 90
    technique. *See* training technique
    volume 85-89
pulling exercises. *See* upper-body pulling exercises
pulling patterns 72-73
pushing exercises. *See* upper-body pushing exercises
pushing patterns 72, 73f

Q

quadraplex 110-111

R

radioulnar 28f
range of motion (ROM). *See* mobility
recovery 85, 89
REM breathing (resistance exercise method) 64-65
repetitions 86, 87t
ROM (range of motion). *See* mobility
rotary motion 55
routines versus programs 81-82
rowing exercises
    cable one-arm horizontal row 234-235
    cable one-arm median row 224-225
    dumbbell horizontal row 232-233
    dumbbell median row 222-223
    machine median row 220-221
running mechanics and speed 44-45

S

sagittal plane. *See* median plane movement
SAID principle 56
sarcomere 11f
scapular 22f, 25f
sensorimotor system 39. *See also* control system
sequence 85, 90
sets and volume 88
shoulder
    cable shoulder extension 226-227
    cable shoulder external rotation 238-239
    dumbbell shoulder external rotation 240-241
    frontal plane movement 26f
    horizontal plane movement 28f
    median plane movement 23f
shrug 236-237
skeleton 4, 5f, 6, 38

slow-twitch muscle fibers 41
speed
    joint mobility and stability and 43-44
    overview 41-42
    relationship with strength 42-43
    running mechanics and 44-45
spinal cord
    described 15-16
    extension 71
    flexion 70
    optimal posture 58, 59f
    positioning of 57
spindles, muscle 16
split routines 94, 100-103
squat patterns 73-74
squats
    balance 142-143
    barbell 148-149
    body weight 140-141
    narrow-stance 146-147
    wide-stance 144-145
stability 34-36
stabilization 60-62
stabilizer muscles 13
strength
    genetics and 31
    muscle size and 31
    relationship with speed 42-43
    tempo and 33
    transfer of 32
    types of 31-32
stretching and mobility 39-41, 46
supine trunk rotation 128-129
swiss ball-based exercises
    double-leg hip flexion 168-169
    dumbbell one-arm horizontal press 202-203
    reverse trunk flexion 120-121
    trunk extension 124-125
    trunk flexion 116-117
synergist muscles 12-13
synovial joints 6
system of naming exercises 106

T
tempo 62-63, 87
trainer techniques
    balance squat 143
    barbell hang clean 161
    barbell hip extension 173
    barbell horizontal press 201
    barbell scapular elevation 237
    barbell squat 149
    basic instruction requirements 65-66
    bent-leg raises 113
    body weight squat 141
    body weight stationary lunge 153
    braced one-leg hip flexion 167
    cable hip abduction 177
    cable hip adduction 179
    cable knee extension 181
    cable knee flexion 185
    cable one-arm 90-degree elbow extension 215
    cable one-arm 90-degree elbow flexion 245
    cable one-arm decline horizontal press 205
    cable one-arm frontal pull-down 231
    cable one-arm horizontal row 235
    cable one-arm median row 225
    cable shoulder extension 227
    cable shoulder external rotation 239

cable trunk rotation with flexion 133
cable trunk rotation with press 137
cable trunk rotation with pull 135
cable zero-degree elbow extension 217
dumbbell 15-degree elbow flexion 243
dumbbell frontal press 211
dumbbell horizontal press 199
dumbbell horizontal row 233
dumbbell incline median press 209
dumbbell median row 223
dumbbell one-arm/one-leg frontal press 213
dumbbell one-leg ankle extension 189
dumbbell one-leg hip extension 175
dumbbell reverse lunge 155
dumbbell shoulder external rotation 241
dumbbell side lunge 157
dumbbell snatch 163
dumbbell swiss ball one-arm horizontal press 203
45-degree hip extension 171
four-point core activation 109
half ball trunk lateral flexion 127
incline bench reverse trunk flexion 119
incline bench trunk extension 123
incline bench trunk flexion 115
machine ankle flexion 195
machine bent-leg ankle extension 193
machine frontal pull-up 229
machine knee extension 183
machine knee flexion 187
machine median row 221
machine seated leg press 151
machine straight-leg ankle extension 191
machine trunk rotation 131
med ball traveling lunge 159
narrow-stance squat 147
quadraplex 111
squat rack decline push-up 207
supine trunk rotation 129
swiss ball double-leg hip flexion 169
swiss ball reverse trunk flexion 121
swiss ball trunk extension 125
swiss ball trunk flexion 117
wide-stance squat 145
training phases 91-93
training technique
    alignment 56-57
    breathing 63-65
    exercise motion 55-56
    goal identification 54-55
    positioning 57-60
    stabilization 60-62
    tempo 62-63
    trainer techniques. See trainer techniques
translatory motion 55
transrotational motion 55
trunk
    cable trunk rotation with flexion 132-133
    cable trunk rotation with press 136-137
    cable trunk rotation with pull 134-135
    frontal plane movement 24f
    half ball trunk lateral flexion 126-127
    horizontal plane movement 27f

incline bench reverse trunk flexion 118-119
    incline bench trunk extension 122-123
    incline bench trunk flexion 114-115
    machine trunk rotation 130-131
    median plane movement 22f
    rotation 71, 72f
    steps when selecting exercises 107
    supine trunk rotation 128-129
    swiss ball reverse trunk flexion 120-121
    swiss ball trunk extension 124-125
    swiss ball trunk flexion 116-117

U
upper-body pulling exercises
    barbell scapular elevation 236-237
    cable one-arm 90-degree elbow flexion 244-245
    cable one-arm frontal pull-down 230-231
    cable one-arm horizontal row 234-235
    cable one-arm median row 224-225
    cable shoulder extension 226-227
    cable shoulder external rotation 238-239
    dumbbell 15-degree elbow flexion 242-243
    dumbbell horizontal row 232-233
    dumbbell median row 222-223
    dumbbell shoulder external rotation 240-241
    machine frontal pull-up 228-229
    machine median row 220-221
    steps when selecting exercises 219
upper-body pushing exercises
    barbell horizontal press 200-201
    cable one-arm 90-degree elbow extension 214-215
    cable one-arm decline horizontal press 204-205
    cable zero-degree elbow extension 216-217
    dumbbell frontal press 210-211
    dumbbell horizontal press 198-199
    dumbbell incline median press 208-209
    dumbbell one-arm/one-leg frontal press 212-213
    dumbbell swiss ball one-arm horizontal press 202-203
    squat rack decline push-up 206-207
    steps when selecting exercises 197

V
$\dot{V}O_2$max (maximal oxygen consumption) 33
volume
    defined 85-86
    duration 88
    frequency 88-89
    intensity and 83-84
    repetitions 86, 87t
    sets 88
    tempo and 87

W
wrist
    frontal plane movement 26f
    median plane movement 23f

About the Author

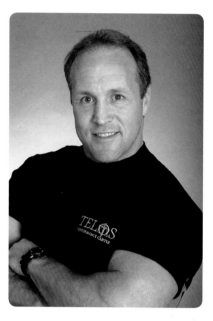

Everett Aaberg has been both a teacher and practitioner of resistance training for more than 15 years. He is currently the director of fitness services and co-owner of the TELOS Fitness Center in Dallas, Texas. A highly sought international presenter and consultant, Aaberg provides continuing education services for several fitness organizations and health clubs around the United States. He also serves as an instructor for the Cooper Institute, where his books are used for two of their most popular courses, The Biomechanics of Resistance Training and Optimal Performance Training.

Aaberg has been a certified personal trainer through some of the most highly accredited organizations in the United States, including the American Council on Exercise (ACE), the American College of Sports Medicine (ACSM), and the National Academy of Sports Medicine (NASM). He is also a certified strength and conditioning specialist through the National Strength and Conditioning Association (NSCA). Aaberg was recognized as an IDEA Personal Trainer of the Year and has been regularly selected by industry and trade magazines as one of the top trainers in the United States.

Aaberg holds a bachelor's degree in exercise sciences and recreation management with continuing education in exercise physiology, anatomy, kinesiology, biomechanics, and nutrition. He was a collegiate academic All-American in football and has won several state and national powerlifting championships and bodybuilding titles, including Amateur Athletic Union (AAU) and National Physique Committee (NPC) Mr. Colorado titles and the Mr. Junior America title.

Aaberg lives in Dallas, Texas, and trains at the TELOS Fitness Center.